# Breaking the Yeast Curse:
## *Food and Unconditional Love for Magic Healing*

*By Dr. Juliet Tien*
*D. N. Sc., M. S. N., B. S. N., R. N., C. S.*

**Infinite Success International**
**Publishing House**
**Las Vegas, Nevada**

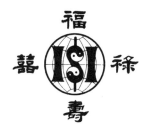

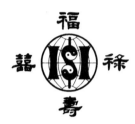

**Second Printing: July 2000**

**Other Books authored by Dr. Juliet Tien and published by ISI Publishing House:**
*Healthy & Tasty: Dr. J's Anti-Yeast Cooking*
*Being the Best You Can Be: A Practical Guide for Harmony and Prosperity*
Ordering Department: 1-800-715-3053

Library of Congress Catalog Card Number: 97-93149

ISBN: 1-89042-01-4

*Printed in the United States of America*

# Dedication

This book is dedicated to all those who helped me survive severe yeast disorders in my early years. It is also dedicated to my clients, who have constantly enhanced my knowledge and effectiveness in treating yeast disorders by sharing their joys and agonies with me in the healing process.

# Preface

The information contained in this book may generate "Aha" among readers who have experienced yeast disorder symptoms at one time or the other, to a greater or lesser degree. It may also raise some eyebrows, especially among traditional health professionals. The message I have been trying to convey to the public in the past through newspaper articles, radio talk shows, television shows, and numerous speeches in national and international conferences is very clear: **yeast disorder is associated with all diseases!** Attention Deficit Disorder (ADD), Acquired Immune Deficiency Syndrome (AIDS), allergies, arthritis, cancer, Chronic Fatigue Syndrome (CFS), depression, diabetes, Epstein-Barr virus, impotence, mononucleosis, phobias, Premenstrual Syndrome (PMS), prostate problems, weight problems, etc., are all associated with yeast overgrowth in your body. Once you employ a holistic approach to treating yeast disorders and related illnesses, you will regain your balance physically, mentally and spiritually.

Whether you agree with me or not, just follow some of my suggestions in the book for at least three months and record the progress. You may be surprised by the amount of increased energy, mental clarity and productivity you will experience! We are all living and dying at the same time. The benefits you get from the anti-yeast approach in this book will help you live or die more comfortably.

Although I have more than 21 years of formal education, the knowledge and skills I share with you in this book are purely experiential. At the present time, no formal curriculum on yeast disorder symptoms and treatments is being offered in any medical, nursing, acupuncture nor chiropractic schools in the United States or abroad. Licensed health professionals and paraprofessionals are sadly lacking in practical knowledge and skills in yeast disorder treatment. If you are a health professional and allow yourself to learn something from this book, numerous clients of yours will benefit as a result of this knowledge.

The good news is that the general public as a whole are increasingly aware of the necessity to change dietary habits. This awareness has caused the springing up of many health food stores in the United States and all over the world. Although the food items carried in health food stores are not perfect according to my "Eight Commandments," there has been a tremendous increase of yeast-free foods in the past few years. The public's demand of yeast-free foods has even prompted supermarkets and pharmacies to carry a few items. "Anti-yeast living" is now becoming a trend, not a fad!

Anti-yeast living is not only important for human beings, it is also important for animals. More than 50% of dogs over 50 pounds die of some form of cancer. The Colorado State University Veterinary Hospital is considered the best in the country. However, their treatment methods are conventional: surgery, chemotherapy and radiation -- the same as those for humans. Follow the anti-yeast cooking in my book, *Healthy and Tasty* and feed your dogs or cats yeast-free foods -- the same way you should feed yourself. Remember, in the good old days, pets ate human food before canned food became available. Give your pets a chance to be healthy and to increase longevity!

As you can see, much work needs to be done to educate the general public, the health professionals and the food industries, not just for the sake of humans but for animals as well. I alone cannot do it all. A Chinese proverb says, "tossing the brick to induce jade." Hopefully, this book can serve as a "wake-up call" for many and thus generate necessary activities to "clean house" on all levels. If we all are conscious of anti-yeast living, our health expenditures will be reduced by manifolds!

6

# Acknowledgments

To my daughter, Melisa Tien,
    an English major at UCLA who edited part of this book during her
    holiday break.
To my son, Charles Tien, an accounting major at USC,
    who edited part of this book and provided invaluable support to make
    the completion of this book possible.
To my mother, Chou-Chi Lee,
    who gave much help with housework which enabled me to finish this
    book within the least possible time.
To my deceased father, Fang Lee,
    who left me with many legacies including hard work and tenacity
    necessary for a challenging task such as writing a book.
To my friend, Gordon Hyatt,
    who edited early versions of this book three years ago.
To my friend, Roger Lindmark,
    who encouraged me to finish this book.
To my friend, Urbara Scott,
    who provided valuable editorial comments and showed much faith
    in me and my work.
To my friend, Jocelyn Tung,
    who offered emotional and financial support at the crucial time.
To Bruni Pelletier,
    who meticulously proofread this book and loyally met deadlines.
To my clients,
    who trusted my knowledge and skills in treating yeast disorders, and
    survived the physical and mental detoxification processes.
To the universe,
    which gave me an opportunity to experience how it was like to be ill,
    and how to help people get well based on that firsthand experience.

I thank you all wholeheartedly!

# Table of Contents

# Part I

# The Yeast Curse

# Chapter 1

# Born with the Curse

———◆———

*Typhoon,* a strong rain and wind storm was sweeping the entire island. "The Beautiful Island" (Formosa) was terribly battered. Tree branches broke and the country roads were flooded.

In a little clay house, the flame of an oil lamp was swirling back and forth each time the strong wind seeped through the seams in between the clay blocks. The shadows of the furniture were also swirling back and forth with the oil lamp flame which made the little clay house even spookier. A young woman was sitting next to a rectangular, wooden fruit box, crying. The bottom of the wooden box was padded with hay and on top of the hay laid a female infant's body. The infant had stopped breathing and the young mother was crying helplessly.

Shortly after World War II, many infants did not survive tetanus due to poor hygiene. A typical way to cut the umbilical cord when a baby was born was to smash a ceramic rice bowl, boil a sharp-edged broken piece for the purpose of disinfection and then use that as a scissor to cut the cord. The young woman thought that her firstborn had met with an ill fate as had many babies in the poor village. Worst of all, when the babies did not survive, they were usually dumped in the long, big river because there were no funds or lands to bury them.

A next-door neighbor got up in the middle of the night to go to the outhouse. He heard that the woman was crying so he knocked at the wooden door. After he listened to the woman's explanation, he found out that the woman was alone. Her in-laws were out of town and her husband was being imprisoned by Chiang Kai-shek's regime because his friends' friends were involved in resisting the new government which had just been expelled from mainland China by the communists. The neighbor quickly felt the baby's body and found out that its body temperature was still quite warm. That was a sign of hope to him. He urged the young woman to take the seemingly dead baby and to hail a hooded tricycle.

The three of them and the tricycle peddler moved slowly but surely through the storm toward an infant doctor's clinic in town. They paid a visit to the most famous pediatrician in the small town. The western-trained pediatrician gave the baby some kind of injection that brought the baby back to life. However, he was not sure that the baby would eventually survive. According to the Chinese custom, when a baby was difficult to raise, he or she should be adopted by a Chinese doctor to break the curse. Thrilled by the fact that the baby was alive, the young woman quickly found a famous Chinese doctor in town and had her baby adopted by him. Since then the baby had been raised on Chinese herbs.

**That sickly baby was me and the young woman was my mother. The neighbor, the pediatrician and my Godfather have long been deceased. Obviously the curse was broken, since I am still alive today!**

What I suffered from was a case of severe yeast disorders. When I look back, I realize that I was born with yeast disorders since my mother was under a tremendous amount of stress during her pregnancy because of the fact that Taiwan was bombed out of shape during World War II and the villagers were suffering from famine and starvation immediately afterwards. Furthermore, my father had been imprisoned by Chiang Kai-shek's regime for several months during my mother's pregnancy and after the childbirth.

She herself had a bad case of yeast disorders because of the stress, poor nutrition and poor hygiene. Bingo! I was born with the yeast curse!

> **Being raised on Chinese herbs had sustained my life. However, the quality of my life was far from being great. I suffered from a cluster of symptoms of a severe case of yeast disorder. Basically, the symptoms were present from head to toe.**

The most devastating symptom was frequent migraine headaches. I remember many sleepless nights when I was in elementary school. I tossed back and forth in bed trying to find a comfortable position to get some sleep with, no luck. The shooting pain shifted from one side of my head to another no matter how I positioned myself. The following day I would be exhausted from lack of sleep. Chronic Fatigue Syndrome had set in. Consequently, I could not concentrate on my schoolwork and my grades fluctuated.

Part of my head symptoms was sinus congestion. My sinuses were often so clogged that I could not breathe. As a result, I was not getting enough oxygen and my head was always foggy. When I was in high school, I used part of my scholarship money to see a western trained ENT (Eye, Nose and Throat) doctor. He diagnosed that I had a deviated septum. He recommended surgery for correction. I did not have enough money for surgery, so he gave me some drug in a tablet form which was supposed to nourish my brain and to eliminate my fatigue and foggy mind. It did not work the way the ENT doctor claimed. Instead, I was extremely sleepy all the time. I had to stop taking the brain pills after a week of struggling to be awake. His next strategy was using an electric burner to burn off the swelling tissue in my nostrils so that I would have a wider passage in my nose for the air to travel through. Not only did this treatment not work, it also caused sneezing and bleeding when the charcoaled scar tissue began to fall off.

Sore throat was another head symptom. During the New Year holidays, the Chinese usually gave or received boxes of candies and cookies as gifts. Being a sugar addict at that time, I often ate a whole tall can of candies in a day. By the end of the day, my throat was so sore that I could not even swallow water. Aside from holidays, I also ate lots of sugary Chinese pastries. If there was nothing particular to eat, I would just eat a big chunk of brown sugar. The end result was, of course, frequent sore throats.

The most annoying symptom for me at that time was the acne! During my junior high school years, my face was covered by large, pus-filled pimples. Every morning I spent a lot of time in front of a mirror trying to squeeze out the pus. Of course, that only made it worse! Based on the recommendation of my Godfather and my maternal grandmother (a folk healer), my mother searched all over town for a special herb called "pheasant tail grass" which was supposed to lower my "liver fire" (anxiety), and thus cure my cystic acne. This herb had to be grown in a well or on the shaded side of a hill in order to be effective to correct my problem. When I look back, I realize that I had too much yang chi (anxiety) and it required substance with yin quality to neutralize it. Luckily, through much prayer to Kuan-Yin Buddhisattva (a female Buddha), my mother bumped into a woman who just harvested a whole bunch of pheasant tail grass from a shaded (yin) side of a hill. I don't remember how long I pinched my nose and gagged on that dark-colored potion before my acne disappeared. However, I'm surely glad that they are now history!

My chest was also very vulnerable. I often contracted severe chest colds which lasted several weeks to months. The major cold symptoms were cough and pus-filled mucus. Sometimes I coughed so hard that I had to use my hands to hold my rib cage to reduce spasms and pain. During those coughing attacks, sleep deprivation was a natural result. Needless to say, that was another reason for my poor mental concentration and chronic fatigue.

My digestive system was in total disarray from frequent overeating. Taiwanese were very festive. The first and the fifteenth of every month were routine ancestor worship days. During such days every family would usually prepare extra amounts of fancy foods for their ancestors to enjoy. Since our ancestors would only "eat" these foods spiritually, the living people were the ones who actually devoured these foods right after the worshiping ceremony.

In addition to the twice-a-month overeating routine, Taiwanese also had holidays almost every month. After the New Year's Day, there were Lantern Festival in mid-January, Grave-Cleaning Day in March, Double-

Five Day in May, Double-Seven (Lovers) Day early in July, Ghost-Feeding Day late in July, Moon Festival in August, Nourishing-the-Winter Day in October, and End-of-Year Day in November. Moreover, every little town had its own once-a-year gigantic festival for worshipping their beloved and trusted goddess, Ma Tsu.

In such festivals, I remembered that my family usually set up more than 10 rounded tables to feed more than 100 invited guests each time. Needless to say, I had plenty of opportunities and excuses to overeat all the time! After each overeating episode, I often could smell and taste the sour foods fermenting in my stomach. As a result, I suffered from frequent stomachaches, bloatedness and weight problems.

My body often ached, especially when the weather was damp. Many times when the weatherman announced on the radio that we were going to have a beautiful day, I would scream, "That's a lie!" because my whole body ached. Sure enough, the following morning might have some sunshine, but by the afternoon, the wind blew and the rained poured. My body had become the most accurate weather predictor! I remember being awakened by joint pains in the middle of the night. So I pounded hard on my joints, arms and legs to get some relief. Sometimes I splashed a good portion of rubbing alcohol on my extremities and then massaged them inch by inch. This would give me moments of relief.

I also had a bad case of eczema and athlete's foot. I often had to use a handkerchief to wipe my palms dry; otherwise, the perspiration would worsen the eczema and more itchy water pockets would form on my palms and fingertips. Sometimes I had to smear a layer of white powder that my mother gave to me to heal the raw, open areas on my skin. At one time the athlete's foot was so bad that I could not wear shoes to go to school. I had to wear slippers. During those days, my mother had me soak my feet in a basin of warm water with sulfate in it. This resembled the water from a hot spring which was supposed to be very soothing and healing for any skin diseases. Somehow it helped.

> **Living with illnesses had become a way of life for me. However, one thing I could never adapt to well was the fact that my grades fluctuated.**

From the time I was very little, I was often praised as one of the brightest kids in the classroom. Sometimes my mind was very clear and I had a photographic memory. During such times I easily got the top grades and my academic performance was usually recognized and praised. Other times my head was very foggy. My mental concentration was poor. My body was dragging and I was depressed. During those times, I could not comprehend or retain the materials taught in the classroom no matter how hard I tried. Consequently, my grades suffered, and so did my self-esteem! One of the biggest blows hit me when I did not do well on the "entrance exam."

In Taiwan during that time, in order to attend junior high school, the elementary school graduates must pass a very tough exam called the "entrance exam." The scores one received from the exam would determine what school he or she could attend. For girls, the First Girls' Middle School was the first choice, the Second Girls' Middle School, the second. Since I was number one in my class and number eight in the entire graduating class when I graduated from the large elementary school with thousands of students, everyone (including myself) assumed that I would have an easy time getting into the first-choice school. The result was disappointing! My scores fell into the Second Girls' Middle School. My ego was terribly bruised, but I knew what had happened. During the exam I had one of those blackout-like episodes in which I was not able to concentrate and think well.

The same problem continued in the junior and senior high schools. Even though my efforts were consistent, my grades were not. As a result, I missed out the opportunity to be advanced to the top-choice university without the entrance exam. That was another blow to my ego! Fortunately, I was able to get good enough scores to enter the National Taiwan University in Taipei, Taiwan which was the equivalent of Harvard University in the United States. In a way I was lucky to be able to pull through. The entrance exam was so competitive in Taiwan that it caused a high rate of teenage suicide. When I look back, I wonder how many young kids were suffering from the same illness I had without knowing what was going on.

Another annoying problem was my weight. In elementary and junior high schools, despite the periodic physical illnesses, I was still able to remain physically active. For example, I was a member of the track and field team in junior high. However, by the time I entered senior high school, I lost my stamina and gained a lot of weight. The worst time I had was when I was 50 pounds overweight. Life was depressing for me because I failed to see the purpose of it! At that time the term "yeast disorder" was not coined yet, and nobody (including myself) knew what I was suffering!

Then, one day, my fate changed! While attending a girls school, there was hardly any chance to meet any of the "opposite sex." Also in those days, good girls were not supposed to mingle with boys. However, since sexual hormones began to pump through the bodies of teenagers, the desire to attract the opposite sex was there regardless of the societal norm.

> **Even though I had a fat body at that time, I did have a pretty face (as people would tell me) after my cystic acne was cured. One Sunday afternoon, however, my pretty face was forced to look at my ugly body!**

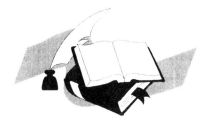

# Chapter 2

# Breaking the Curse

———◆———

*Summer* could be very lovely on the subtropical island. One of the favorite activities for teenagers was to ride on bicycles strolling around town and bathe themselves in the warm sunshine and the balmy breeze. It was one of those enjoyable Sunday afternoons when I bumped into my uncle and his friends during a bicycle ride. My youngest uncle was only three years older than I was and was attending the Chien-Kuo High School (the best boys high school in the nation) at that time. I was excited to have an opportunity to meet my uncle's schoolmates -- a bunch of boys! While he was introducing me to his friends, he said smilingly, "This is the little pig in my family!" He thought he was joking, but I took it very seriously. In fact I was extremely hurt. I went home crying alone for hours.

When I finally stopped crying, I made a vow, "I'm going to change my fate! I'm sick and tired of being sick and tired! I'm going to lose weight and look good!" This was the summer of 1964.

> **Since I was a young kid, I had learned the fact that "if one wants to be successful, just follow the footsteps of those who are already successful."  So, I began to observe people.  There were thin Chinese people and there were fat Chinese people.  I wondered what made them different.**

Pretty soon I figured out one interesting phenomenon:  thin Chinese people tended to be the people from southern China who relied on rice as the main grain; while fat Chinese people tended to be the people from northern China who relied on wheat as the main grain.  I began to wean myself from eating the wheat products such as "Bau Tsu" and "Mang Toa" (wheat dumplings), "Mein" (wheat noodles), and all the wheat breads, wheat cookies, Chinese wheat pancakes,  and so forth and so on.  Instead, I began to eat more rice products.  Luckily, being a Taiwanese, it was not difficult to find rice products such as rice noodles,  Chinese rice cakes and rice pastries.  Several months into my new eating habits, I noticed that my clothes began to hang loose around my waistline.  I was losing weight!

The excitement of this success prompted me to continue my secret experiment.  Knowing that heavy sugar consumption would give me a horrible sore throat, I began to wean myself from sugar as well.  Although there was hidden sugar in a lot of foods, I consciously avoided candies and brown sugar -- they used to be my all-time favorite!  Then I noticed my weight dropped some more!

Slowly but surely, I discovered that weaning myself from dairy, yeast, alcohol and caffeine were also helpful in reducing my weight. Some interesting side benefits were that my mind was getting more consistently clear; I was able to breathe better; I had more energy; I was not always as bloated as I used to be; I experienced less headaches and less episodes of painful and itchy eczema; and most of all, I felt more like a human being! For the first time I felt my head was well planted on my body!

This was a lonely and lengthy process. From 1964 to 1966 (the year I graduated from high school), I lost quite a bit of weight. I began to see curves on my body. However, I was still plump. The following four years in the university, I experienced some minor ups and downs, but for the most part, I continued to lose kilos and inches. The most significant transformation during those four years was psychological in nature. This included defining the purpose and directions in my life, releasing a lot of anger and resentment toward my parents and stabilizing my identity and image.

As mentioned previously, I marginally made entry into the National Taiwan University with the 1966 entrance exam. Even though it was good for my ego that I was in the top university at that time, I was not satisfied with the fact that my scores placed me in the School of Nursing instead of the School of Pharmacy which was my first choice. Since I had been raised on herbs, I always had the ambition to use pharmaceutical technology to advance the use of herbs for human health.

The university policy allowed transfer to a desired department if the student had outstanding academic performance for the first year. I worked extremely hard during my first year in the School of Nursing. Consequently, I got the highest grades in the class and was eligible to transfer to either the School of Pharmacy or the School of Medicine. I was then faced with a very difficult decision. The whole society in Taiwan was status conscious. A medical doctor held more prestige than a pharmacist or a nurse and a pharmacist was regarded as superior to a nurse. After having a taste of the nursing career, I knew that among the three disciplines, nursing was the best one to allow me to work with people. From my observation, the medical doctors were often too busy to mingle with patients, and the pharmacists usually worked with drugs behind the counter, not directly with patients. My true love was to work with people on both physical and psychological aspects. The only field that would satisfy my need and desire was psychiatric/mental health nursing! So, I stayed in the School of Nursing for another three years.

Once the decision was made, I launched a vigorous study of body, mind and spirit. I was like a sponge soaking in a lot of knowledge, skill and experience to prepare myself to be a good psychiatric/mental health nurse. This was the time I was reintroduced to Buddhism. As a kid, I was raised in an environment where my paternal side of the family mostly believed in Taoism and my maternal side of the family strictly believed in Buddhism. Most families believed in both Buddhism and Taoism and had hard times telling the difference between the two. After joining the Buddhist Society at the National Taiwan University, I had an opportunity to learn what Buddhism was all about. I had learned that Buddhism was actually a school of philosophy and a way of life. It was not a religion as most people would think. Since then my life was basically guided by the philosophy and doctrine of Buddhism. This has enabled me to understand the rule of karma (cause-effect relationship) and reincarnation (multiple lives).

I was enlightened by this understanding. I began to understand why I suffered so much since the time I was born. There was a purpose. Although I was not very clear about the exact purpose of these experiences, I knew that as time went by, things would unfold slowly but surely. Consequently, I stopped feeling sorry for myself. I knew that if I wanted to see positive results, I had to plant positive seeds. I was the one who was in charge of my destiny, my karma!

The understanding of karma also helped me release anger and resentment toward my parents. For a while I felt ashamed of my undereducated parents. They both had received only elementary school education during the Japanese occupation. Consequently, they did not even speak Mandarin. They spoke only Taiwanese and Japanese. I used to envy my classmates whose parents were well educated and sophisticated. When I saw a classmate hooking her arm into her father's as they shopped in the open market where my parents and I sold vegetables, my heart ached with envy. I felt deprived of that fatherly love. My father was a farmer and a small merchant working hard all the time to make ends meet. My mother assisted my father to support the family of five children. No time and no money for leisure! I felt deprived and stuck!

After I understood that we each brought karma with us when we were born in order to learn the lessons we had to learn, I began to come to terms with my fate! I realized that my parents had their karma to live through and I shared the common karma with them because I had to learn certain lessons in order for me to grow and expand. I began to look at the positive sides of my parents' lives and behavior. I was amazed to find out that my father, despite being undereducated, was a leader in our community! He was the chief of the "volunteer police" who patrolled the community during theft-active seasons such as Chinese New Year. As a result of his effort, the early morning theft (between 1:00 a.m. and 5:00 a.m.) during the holidays was greatly reduced. Even though he had a hot temper, he was well liked by people in the village.

My mother, even though never formally trained, was a good cook, good seamstress and a good farmer. She was also known to be very kind and generous to other people.

---

**Slowly but surely, I began to discover the legacy my parents had left for me. As a result, my anger and resentment were gradually replaced with appreciation and respect. They were the "nameless heroes!"**

---

As I began to appreciate my parents, I also began to appreciate myself. For years I used to believe that I was short and not attractive. After I entered the university, despite the fact that I was still working on my weight, I often got the comments that I was pretty, petite, cute and talented. Slowly but surely, I allowed these praises to sink in and to work for me. Consequently, I began to blossom. Some of my notable achievements were: frequent appearances of my articles in the medical journal published by the students and faculty at the National Taiwan University College of Medicine; produced, directed and acted in three comedy shows to welcome the new students; and most all, in 1968 co-founded the first community mental health center in Taiwan. These activities had helped establish my image as a multifaceted and multitalented individual. The most satisfying part was that I realized I was a resource to the community and I was making a contribution to society!

My favorite activities during those trying years were walking, hiking, bicycling and swimming. These healthy activities helped keep my mind and body active and in good balance. I also learned how to meditate. That was one of the most beneficial things I ever learned in my life. Meditating daily for 20 to 30 minutes helped me focus on my goals and maintain a positive attitude.

By 1970, when I graduated from the National Taiwan University School of Nursing, I had shed a total of 50 pounds. I began to look like a model. In fact, my aunt was a model at that time, and I often inherited fancy clothes from her. It took me a total of six years to accomplish that! Since then, I have maintained my measurements at 34-24-34 for the past 25 years except the two times I was pregnant with my children! To this day, I can still fit into my 25-year-old miniskirts nicely. Being free of yeast-disorder symptoms, people say that I look 15 years younger than my age. Yes, I look young and I feel young. I look sexy and I feel sexy. The curse was finally broken and remains that way for good!

> **What did it take to break the curse? As you can see, it was the combination of the anti-yeast nutritional program, Chinese herbal therapy, stress management, deep emotional releasing, regular exercise and learning to accept and love yourself and others, especially your parents!**

By sharing my story with you, I am basically "tossing the brick to induce jade." The chapters that follow will give you a more in-depth discussion on symptoms of yeast disorders, their causes and treatments.

# Part II

# Are You Suffering from the Yeast Curse?

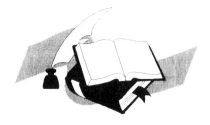

# Chapter 3

# The Missing Diagnosis

———◆———

*If* there was a condition that has been misdiagnosed and improperly treated by most medical professionals, yeast infections are at the top of the list. Many yeast infection symptoms have been mistaken by the medical profession as bacterial or viral infections and consequently have been treated with antibiotics which only make the matters worse.

*Mary, for example, had suffered from severe stomach pain for years. She was a 35-year-old divorcee with two teenage children. Her ex-husband did not provide any child support so she had to work hard to make ends meet. Consequently, she harbored some resentment toward her ex-husband. She enjoyed her career as a personal manager for celebrities, but her working hours were too long for her to enjoy her own life. Her favorite foods were wheat and dairy products, especially cheese. In addition to the symptom of stomach pain, she also experienced constipation, weight gain, poor mental concentration, mood swings, depression, anxiety, shortness of breath, fatigue and aches and pains in her neck and shoulders. She had consulted with many physicians and was subjected to numerous tests. The tests revealed that there was no physical basis for her ailments. Consequently, her primary physician prescribed tagamet for her stomachaches and valium for her anxiety. He also recommended psychotherapy for her depression. Mary tried all these treatment modalities without any results. She began to wonder whether she was a hypochondriac or perhaps something was really wrong with her head!*

*After she was put on an anti-yeast nutritional program and Chinese herbal therapy for a few weeks, her stomachaches greatly reduced. The most important change she made was abstaining from wheat and dairy products. Through psychological counseling, she learned how to effectively release anger and resentment toward her ex-husband. She also learned how to reorganize her daily routine so that she could spend more time with her children, and most of all, leave some time for herself to relax and enjoy life.*

Jill had quite a dramatic experience.

*Jill had her thyroid removed when she was 48 years old due to a malignant tumor. Two years prior to that, she found out that her husband had a love affair with his co-worker. Even though the marriage was saved, she felt the resentment of being betrayed and the fear of being abandoned. After the thyroid surgery, she began to experience symptoms of bloatedness, hair loss, shortness of breath, constipation, high blood pressure, water retention, anxiety, depression, insomnia and extreme fatigue. She had also gained 50 pounds in two years. She was on synthroid to regulate her thyroid hormone. She was also on all sorts of medication for various symptoms without relief. Her thyroid doctor told her that she would have to live with all these symptoms for the rest of her life since she did not have a thyroid gland.*

*She felt so miserable that she became suicidal. On one Christmas Eve, she was lying on the couch crying and praying for God to end her life or bring her hope. Then the doorbell rang. The mailman brought her mail, among which there was a magazine with an article written by me addressing the holistic approach to weight control. In the article I also discussed how to regenerate the thyroid in order to reduce weight effectively. She was so excited to read the article because no other weight loss programs she was exposed to really addressed the thyroid problem. She quickly picked up the phone and left a message on the answering machine in my office to request an emergency appointment.*

*Shortly after the Christmas holidays, she started the anti-yeast therapy which included an anti-yeast nutritional program and Chinese herbal therapy to cleanse the toxins in her system and to regenerate her thyroid function. She was also guided to make peace with her husband. Three months later, somehow a miracle happened. Despite the fact that Jill had a complete thyroid removal, her body began to generate its own thyroxin! As a result, her endocrinologist instructed her to reduce the dosage of synthroid. A few months later, not only did Jill get rid off the symptoms described above, she also lost 50 pounds and looked at least 10 years younger!*

**Yeast disorders do not just affect women. It's equal opportunity for men as well!**

*Rodney, for example, was a 60-year-old man who had suffered from chronic fatigue for many years. Rodney was a light technician in a studio where he often worked long, long hours when he had a job. If the studio was in hiatus, he could go without a job for months. It was either feast or famine. In addition to chronic fatigue, another major symptom was sugar addiction. He craved for sugar all the time so he ate an abundance of candies and sweet fruits. His body and breath had a bad odor which affected his sexual relationship with his wife. He also had frequent temper tantrums. As a result, his wife was so fed up with him that one day she left with a chunk of their lifelong savings. Despite frequent visits to doctors and numerous laboratory tests, Rodney was increasingly fatigued and depressed.*

*When he phoned my office for an appointment, both my secretary and myself had a hard time understanding his speech because he was so weak that he hardly had any strength to talk. After he was instructed to stop eating sugar and concentrated fructose, to take a high dosage of Chinese herbal formulas to cleanse the toxins and body odor, and to release anger toward his wife, he slowly regained his physical and mental strength to deal with his marital crisis.*

---

**Yeast disorders do not discriminate against age either. Children have an easy chance to be affected too.**

---

*Johnny, a three-year-old boy, had suffered from frequent mid-ear infections, sinus congestion, sore throats, short attention span and hyperactivity. In the nursery school, he usually had trouble concentrating and had a hard time finishing a project. He was easily distracted and was easily agitated. His pediatrician put him on antibiotics for his mid-ear infections. Everytime he was on antibiotics, he would feel better and behave better for a short while, but pretty soon the symptoms of earaches would return, and so did the rest of the behavioral problems.*

*On his first visit to my office, Johnny had a hard time sitting still. He was into everything! By the time he left, my office looked like it was hit by a tornado! His parents were instructed to put Johnny on an anti-yeast nutritional program, and to give him Chinese herbal formulas specific to his attention deficit disorder symptoms. Most important of all, his parents and siblings were counseled to maintain harmony and order in the family. In a matter of a few weeks, Johnny behaved like an angel! He proudly told me that his teachers at the nursery school said that he was a smart and handsome boy! In our last session, while his parents were seeing me for therapy, Johnny sat quietly in the same room drawing a picture for me!*

---

**Is there any race or ethnicity immune to yeast disorders? Not a chance!**

---

*Timothy, an Afro-American from Ethiopia had suffered from fatigue, low energy, poor mental concentration, depression and lack of sexual drive. Despite the fact that he was brilliant and well versed, he considered himself an underachiever because he did not have the motivation to pursue his goals in higher education and career advancement. He thought that immigrating to the United States may provide him with an environment to get him motivated so he could move forward. After living in the United States for almost 10 years and being treated for depression and anxiety by western doctors, he found no improvement in his physical and mental conditions.*

*After he was treated with the anti-yeast approach, his mind cleared up, his energy increased and he began to realize how much fear and old baggage he had carried on his shoulders since he was a little kid. This realization enabled him to peel off his unfinished business, layer by layer. For the first time in his life, he was able to breathe more freely and he began to feel like a new man!*

The above cases are typical examples of misdiagnosis and mistreatment of yeast infections. Why are yeast infections so difficult to diagnose and treat by contemporary medical professionals? The answer is very simple: there is no curriculum devoted to yeast disorder diagnosis and treatment in medical trainings. Dr. William Crook's *The Yeast Connection* (1984), Dr. Orian Truss' *The Missing Diagnosis* (1985) and Drs. Trowbridge and Walker's *Yeast Syndrome* (1986) were among the first few publications which began to define the symptoms and treatments for yeast disorders. Even though the term "yeast disorder" was coined by these physicians in the 1980s, most Western-trained doctors still stubbornly believe that the yeast disorder was created by "quack" doctors.

I remember one time when I was on a panel along with another physician to address allergies, a young-looking lady asked us why she had a persistent case of acne. After gathering some information from her regarding other symptoms, I told her that she might have a case of yeast disorder which may be caused by her diet and stress. The physician (cardiologist) on the panel quickly disputed what I said by asserting that yeast disorder symptoms only occur under the breast or in between the toes because of excessive perspiration. He further insisted that it was very common for teenagers to have acne because of hormonal imbalance. The young lady raised her hand and protested, "But, doctor, I'm not a teenager. I'm thirty-six years old!" The audience chuckled. Then the know-it-all doctor replied, "Just try some antibiotics. Tetracycline has been very effective in treating acne!" The omnipotent antibiotics again! In later chapters, you will learn that antibiotics are actually one of the causes for a severe case of yeast disorder!

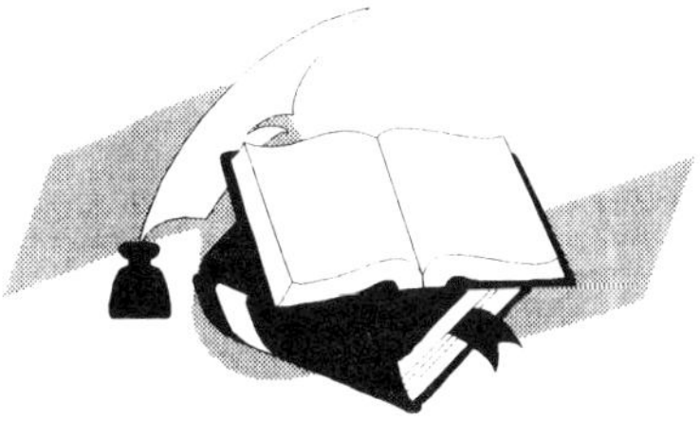

# Chapter 4

# What are Yeasts?

*Fungi* have an extended family. Yeasts belong to the fungus family which consists of at least 100,000 to 250,000 species. They include yeasts, mold, mildew, rots, smuts and mushrooms. The characteristics of fungi is the lack of chlorophyl. Consequently, they cannot perform photosynthesis and are parasitic and saprophytic (feeding off dead organisms).

The function of yeasts is to break down dead bodies so that organic matter can be turned into its basic elements of oxygen, nitrogen, carbon and phosphorus. Without yeasts, we could be in serious trouble because dead bodies of animals and plants would just pile up. We need yeasts to assist in the recycling of ecology.

However, overgrowth of yeasts can also break down living organisms. There are at least 20 to 30 different types of pathogenic yeasts which cause illnesses. Candida is one member of the yeast family. Candida albicans alone has 50 to 60 different strains which cause infections. Consequently, it is no surprise that almost every individual in contemporary society suffers from yeast infections at one time or another, to a greater or lesser degree.

> **Because yeasts normally live on mucous membranes, contemporary laboratory tests such as blood tests, x-rays or stool cultures usually cannot detect their presence.**

Many clients who sought help at my office reported that all the tests performed by their physicians were negative; however, they still felt miserable. Observation of the eyes, skin and tongue and knowledge of a detailed health history are the best ways to determine whether an individual is infected with yeasts.

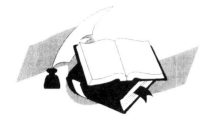

# Chapter 5

# Yeast Disorder Symptoms

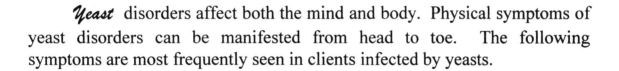

*Yeast* disorders affect both the mind and body. Physical symptoms of yeast disorders can be manifested from head to toe. The following symptoms are most frequently seen in clients infected by yeasts.

### Headaches:
Recurrent and frequent sinus or migraine headaches.

### Mid-ear infections:
Infants and children are very susceptible to mid-ear infections. In most cases, they inherited yeast disorders from their mothers' bloodstream or birth canal.

### Eye Problems:
Irritation of eyes, burning and swelling of eyelids, dryness of eyes or decreased vision.

### Sore Throats:
Recurrent and prolonged sore throats or tonsillitis, difficulty in swallowing.

### Mouth Thrush:
Especially common among people with AIDS (Acquired Immune Deficiency Syndrome) or ARC (AIDS-related complex), or babies.

### Respiratory System:
Bronchitis, pneumonia, asthma, tightness of chest, sinus infections, excessive mucous or post-nasal drip.

### Digestive System:
Bloatedness in stomach and abdomen after eating, indigestion, constipation, diarrhea, ulcerative colitis, food allergies, craving for sugar, cheese, breads, caffeine, nicotine, alcohol or drugs, and inability to lose or gain weight regardless of the amount of food intake.

### Immune System:
Susceptibility to colds, flus, infections and allergies, extreme fatigue and low energy.

### Cardiovascular System:
Sluggish blood circulation, palpitations, cold hands and feet and varicose veins.

### Reproductive System:
Impotence, painful sexual intercourse, vaginal or prostate infections, PMS (Premenstrual Syndrome), vaginal itch, endometriosis and menstrual irregularity.

### Elimination System:
Kidney or bladder infections, hemorrhoids, mucous in stool, anal itch and burning during urination.

### Endocrine System:
Hypothyroidism, hypoglycemia and diabetes mellitus.

### Skin:
Acne, eczema, psoriasis, scaling skin lesions, rashes, athlete's foot, cellulite, inflammation of tips of fingers and toes, hair loss and brittle nails.

*Muscular-skeletal System:*

Aches and pains in muscles and joints, bursitis, stiff and swollen fingers, and pains in the neck, shoulders and back.

---

**When people have a severe case of yeast infection, they may experience a good number of the above physical symptoms. In addition, their eyes may have a sleepy look and tend to blink frequently. Their tongues tend to crack or be coated which is an indication of poor colon function.**

---

In addition to physical symptoms, the following mental/psychological symptoms can also be present:

*Mental Concentration:*
Decreased memory and attention span, feeling foggy or spaced-out, difficulties in concentration and drowsiness.

*Depression:*
Loss of interest in daily life activities, lack of motivation and suicidal thoughts.

*Mood Swings:*
Anger, irritability, frustration and defensiveness.

*Phobias:*
Fear of motion such as elevators, escalators, airplanes, trains, buses or boats, or fear of crowds (agoraphobia or social phobia).

*Anxiety Attacks:*
Inability to handle daily chores, shortness of breath and panic attacks.

*Insomnia:*
Inability to fall asleep or sleep through the night.

# Part III

# Causes of Yeast Disorders

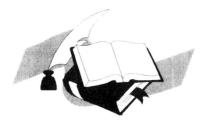

# Chapter 6

# Physical Factors

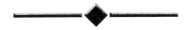

*Poor* eating habits, liberal use of chemicals, lack of exercise and pre-existing illnesses can cause the breakdown of the immune system and the thriving of yeasts.

## Poor Eating Habits:

Sugar, dairy, wheat and yeast products are favorite foods for yeasts. Unfortunately, a great number of people live on these foods. When you feed the right foods to yeasts, they are so happy that they start an instant rock n'and roll party! After having a great time, like any other beings, they have to go to the bathroom. They then use your body as a toilet to dump lots of toxins.

When they suck your energy through their strong, vampire-like hooks, you experience extreme fatigue or lethargy because when you eat, you are actually feeding an extended family in your body. When yeasts deposit toxins, you may suffer from allergy symptoms such as sinus congestion, headaches, arthritis-like aches and pains, lower back pain, bloatedness, constipation, or bladder or kidney infections. Both yeasts and their toxins can clog the liver, pancreas and thyroid and make the metabolism of sugar sluggish. This is one of the causes for hypoglycemia. Hypoglycemia can then contribute to headaches, foggy mind, poor mental concentration, poor memory and irritability. Another factor contributing to your foggy mind is that when yeasts ferment in your body, a by-product, ammonia, can alter your thinking process and cause disorientation.

## Excessive Use of Antibiotics and Other Chemicals:

Chemicals such as antibiotics, cortisone, anti-cancer drugs, anti-AIDS drugs, birth control pills, alcohol, nicotine, caffeine, marijuana, heroin and cocaine can break down the immune system and cause severe yeast disorders.

> **The liberal use of antibiotics and cortisone in recent years has particularly resulted in the widespread occurrence of yeast disorders. When these powerful chemicals get into your body, it's like dropping atomic bombs on Nagasaki and Hiroshima!**

During World War II, after the bombing, all beings in the immediate bombed areas were killed instantly. Guess who came back first? Not cockroaches! The Japanese had a heck of a hard time cleaning up a lot of yeasts in these cities. Giant mushrooms were everywhere. Too bad they were not edible because they were full of radiation!

The chemicals, designed to control infections and inflammations, kill off both bad guys (e.g., bacteria, yeasts, viruses and parasites) and good guys (e.g., friendly bacteria floras). Hence, they create a vacuum upon the initial use. At this time you may experience temporary relief, because there's nobody home; it's nice and quiet. However, this honeymoon time usually does not last long. It takes good guys a long time to recover. However, the bad guys thrive like the weeds after a summer rainfall. A great imbalance is thus created. Consequently, symptoms of yeast disorder worsen each time after treatment with these potent drugs.

## Lack of Exercise:

Some people indulge themselves in the conveniences provided by modern technology. The only exercise they do is walking to and from their cars when they go to work. After work, they often glue themselves to their sofa and become couch potatoes. Lack of exercise can cause poor blood and oxygen supply to the brain. The mind can become foggy and forgetful. Many people mistakenly think they are becoming senile, but their ages don't qualify them for that condition. This symptom can happen at almost any age.

Yeasts love a still environment. When blood circulation is sluggish, they like it better because they have a lesser chance to be flushed out. Body cells and tissues can also be malnourished as a result of poor blood circulation. Consequently, their ability to expel toxins is hampered. This will decrease the functions of major organs such as the heart, liver and kidneys. In a vicious circle, more toxins will be stored in the body, which in turn will further damage the body's ability to cleanse and heal!

## Pre-existing Illnesses:

People who already suffer from illnesses such as cancer, AIDS, multiple sclerosis (MS), lupus, diabetes, etc., have a tendency to contract yeast infections because their immune systems are low during the course of these degenerative diseases. A vicious circle is usually created with the treatment of chemotherapy, radiation, antibiotics, cortisone, and other drugs. People with the above mentioned illnesses tend to be physically inactive or bedridden due to the nature of these illnesses. This, in turn, results in poor blood circulation which consequently allows yeasts to grow. Skin rash, mouth thrush, respiratory tract or urinary tract infections are but a few examples of yeast disorder symptoms associated with these diseases.

Alcoholism is another condition which creates an incubator for yeast overgrowth. The fermentation process makes alcoholic beverages become loaded with yeasts, sugar and chemicals. In addition, alcohol clogs and hardens the liver, which in turn makes the detoxifying function of the liver sluggish. A vicious circle thus begins. An alcoholic husband or wife with yeast disorders can give the infection to the spouse through sexual intercourse. If the wife is pregnant, these yeast infections can then be transmitted to the baby through the bloodstream or birth canal.

---

**Many babies were thus born with yeast disorders which often manifest in symptoms such as colic, recurrent mid-ear infections, sore throats, flus and colds.**

---

The parent's alcoholism is not the only cause for babies to inherit yeast disorders. The aforementioned pre-existing illnesses or other illnesses of the parents can also facilitate yeast overgrowth and make the babies vulnerable to yeast infections.

Excessive use of laxatives or enemas either chemical or herbal can also cause imbalance of bacteria floras in the colon and hence contribute to more yeast overgrowth. In many cases, constipation is associated with yeast infections. Consistent use of laxatives and enemas create a further imbalance and a vicious circle.

Regular use of colonics can also destroy the balance of good bacteria floras in the colon and thus create a good environment for yeast infections. Usually, when people go for colonics, they are either constipated or feel the need to detoxify their systems, or both. Colonics are an exaggerated enema which uses gallons of soap water or other solutions to flush out whatever is stored in the colon, including fecal materials, good and bad bacteria floras and nutrition. Just like dropping an atomic bomb in your body (taking antibiotics), colonics create a vacuum in the lower digestive tract which makes you feel "nice and quiet" for a while. After that honeymoon state, constipation or more toxins build up again. Consequently, you need more colonics in order to feel good again. Despite the fact that many colonic therapists use good bacteria floras such as acidophilus in a suppository, powder, capsule or liquid form to restore the balance in the irrigated colon, the results are usually less than satisfactory. The following is a case example to illustrate this unintended problem:

*Robin, a 22-year-old woman, had been a vegetarian since she was 15 years old. She is always health-minded. She went to the gym to work out five days a week. As a result of her persistent, good performance, she was recruited by the gym as an aerobics instructor. When colonic therapy became popular, Robin incorporated that as part of her health maintenance. She had been getting colonics once a week for three years. In the recent year, she began to suffer from severe constipation, so she opted for more colonics. As a result, her colon became more sluggish. Without strong laxatives or colonics, she was unable to move her bowels.*

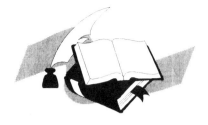

# Chapter 7

# Psychological Factors

———◆———

*Acute* or chronic stress can deplete the immune system, inhibit the growth of friendly bacterial floras and facilitate the overgrowth of yeast. Based on my over 25 years of experience in counseling people from various countries and ethnic groups, I have found that *psychological stress is the primary cause for yeast disorders. Unfinished business, boredom and "Busy-Taking-Care-of-Others Syndrome" are common causes for chronic psychological stress.*

## Unfinished Business:

Frederick Perls (1969, 1975), nicknamed Fritz, a renowned psychiatrist, coined the phrase "unfinished business" or "unfinished situation." This phrase denotes that an individual has been in and out of the emotional garbage pail and does not resolve the inner conflicts. These inner conflicts can stem from relationships with parents, parent surrogates, children, spouses, siblings, friends, relatives, partners and co-workers.

> **When your existence is haunted by unfinished business, you are likely to carry negative emotions such as anger, resentment, grief, regret and guilt.**

When that is the case, you will be slowed down in every aspect of your life. This situation is similar to driving a car with the hand brake on. Although you can move forward if you put extra pressure on the gas pedal, the car (the human body) will endure wear and tear and eventually break down.

An interesting study was done by a nutritional immunologist, Dr. Jau-Fei Chen, in 1991. Every morning when she walked into her laboratory, she used a pencil to strike through the cage housing a few mice. After a few hours, she checked the spleen cell counts of these mice. Their spleen cell counts dropped by 50% because they were distressed by the horrible noise caused by the striking of the pencil. The spleen is responsible for the production of white cells -- members of the army which defends our body. If we are under constant stress, can you imagine how much our immunity would be depleted over time?

People who come from dysfunctional families tend to harbor much anger and resentment. Adult Children of Alcoholics (ACAs) are good examples. ACAs tend to go through a period of chronic stress due to either or both of their parents' emotional unavailabililty, chaos, disharmony and sometimes domestic violence as a result of drinking.

*Arlene, a 21-year-old college student, was taken home from a college on the east coast. She was extremely lethargic and almost catatonic at the time she was escorted to her home in California. She parented her parents for years when they were actively drinking. Her father had had an affair which led to a legal separation from her mother. Her mother had been sober for five years and had been attending AA meetings.*

*Although Arlene's mother began to assume motherly responsibilities in recent years during her sobriety, Arlene experienced extreme fatigue, food allergies, digestive problems, depression, inability to concentrate, weight gain, bad body odor and anxiety attacks. Her symptoms made her angry and frightened because she used to be very energetic, active and popular. She was hospitalized for psychiatric disorders for three weeks without improvement. With the encouragement of a friend who had been successfully treated for similar conditions, Arlene and her mother sought help through a holistic approach.*

## Boredom:

Boredom can slow down both mental and physical activities, and in turn, depress the immune system. When the immune system is sluggish, opportunistic organisms such as yeasts, bacteria, viruses and parasites will have a greater opportunity to take over.

In a cross-cultural study (Tien, 1981 & 1986), I investigated the subject of life satisfaction for the elderly in three cultures. The results indicated that the elderly participants who enjoyed the most life satisfaction were those who had an active physical and mental life. Their inactive counterparts tended to suffer from more physical and psychological ailments such as arthritis, constipation, digestive problems, high cholesterol, hypertension, depression, insomnia, or lethargy.

> **Yeast disorders affect bored people of all ages, not just the elderly.**

The following two cases will help illustrate this cause and effect relationship:

*Stella, a 29-year-old woman, had been through several unfulfilling relationships in the past 10 years. She was always looking, but she did not meet anyone who was ready to make a commitment to a loving and lasting relationship. She was bored with her job because she was overqualified for the work she was doing. She suffered from chronic fatigue for many years and had consulted with numerous physicians, including a holistic chiropractor who treated her with some expensive herbs.*

*Frustrated by the fact that she had spent much money, time and energy on finding a cure for her fatigued body, she finally realized that she also needed psychological counseling to change her lifestyle. After a few weeks of therapy with me, she redefined her career goals and found a new boyfriend who kept her busy and excited. Her chronic fatigue and other yeast disorder symptoms disappeared quickly.*

Betty is another example.

*Betty was 60 years old and had suffered from chronic fatigue all her life. She had worked at the same job for more than 30 years. Although she enjoyed her salary which reflected her seniority, she was bored with the same routine day in and day out. She was very attractive. However, she had never been married and had not been in a relationship for a long time. Her reason was that her energy level only allowed her to go to work, come home, feed the dog, fix some dinner for herself, and then collapse and "go into a coma" until the following morning. After receiving therapy for both physical and psychological cleansing, she began to see the alternatives to a routine life. Her chronic fatigue dissipated quickly.*

## Busy-Taking-Care-of-Others Syndrome:

Some people have developed a habit of taking care of others and neglecting their own welfare. Usually these people knowingly or unknowingly suffer from low self-esteem or insecurity; therefore, they have strong needs to take care of others in order to feel that they are important and wanted. This care-taking behavior is a form of seeking approval. Since they did not get approval from their parents, they turn to other sources for approval.

> **Unfortunately, after spending a good many years helping others, they become physically and mentally fatigued since their real needs are not recognized and met.**

Cary is a good example.

*Cary had suffered for three years from chronic fatigue. Her mother died of cancer when she was five years old. She had a good relationship with her father, but was craving for her mother's love. In order to fill that void, she devoted herself to taking care of others to an extreme. She volunteered in many health organizations such as the American Cancer Society and Red Cross. After she recognized her own needs and began to take steps to meet them, she was able to snap out of chronic fatigue and other symptoms in a matter of a few months.*

Susan, a 46-year-old woman, is another example.

*She had suffered from fatigue, sinus congestion, food allergies, insomnia and earaches for two years. Although she did not work after she was married, she was extremely active in volunteer work. She chaired many major campaigns for some important political figures. She was also very devoted to church activities. She had good relationships with her mother and other family members, but had hellish experiences with her father.*

*Her father was a physician and was very critical of her ever since she could remember. Although she tried very hard to please her father, the conflicts remained unresolved after her father passed away. She was treated by a holistic doctor with an anti-candida diet and acupuncture. Her symptoms lessened but were still present. She finally realized the need to resolve the conflicts with her father spiritually and to take care of herself more diligently than taking care of others.*

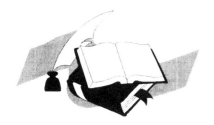

# Chapter 8

# Environmental Factors

◆

*Environmental* factors play a significant role in your health. Yeasts are everywhere. They are in the air you breathe, the water you drink, the carpet you sit on and the furniture you use.

## Air Pollution:

Molds, dust, dirt and flower pollen in the air can facilitate the growth of yeasts. A recent study at Loma Linda University (Pope, 1991) indicates that cancer is linked with smog in southern California. Occasionally you may hear the weatherman say that "the air quality" is poor and the mold count is high today!"

Not only will the polluted air damage the function of your body's sewage system, but the yeasts in the air will also aggravate the growth of the existing yeasts in your body.

## Water Pollution:

A recent study revealed that drinking chlorinated water raises the chance of a person having cancer by 4%. Chemicals in the water you drink can clog your liver and hamper your immune system.

---

**The yeasts and bacteria in the water you drink or the water you use to shower with can cause chronic health problems.**

---

The following is a typical case example:

*Carol, a 32-year-old woman, had suffered from chronic fatigue, bloatedness, alternate constipation and diarrhea, swollen and painful joints and fingers, sinus congestion and migraine headaches for years. She had gone through numerous tests and treatments without results. She suspected that the weather might have something to do with her illness, so she moved her family to a wooded area in Oregon. Although she enjoyed the "clean air," there was no electricity and they had to rely on a well for water supply. Soon she found her symptoms worsened. She hardly could sleep at night because of severe sinus congestion and headaches. Her depression, anxiety and mood swings, especially one or two weeks before her period, had made her marriage very rocky.*

*After the divorce, she moved out of the woods and back to California. All of a sudden she found out that her symptoms improved, although they did not totally dissipate. After taking a careful look at her history, it was found that she used to use a lot of tetracycline for her acne during her late teens. Together with heavy stress from her marital discord and improper diet, she developed a good case of yeast disorder. When she moved to Oregon, the rainy weather, moldy woods and contaminated water made her yeast infections worse. After she moved back to California, a drier weather actually worked in her favor, comparatively speaking.*

## Other Pollution:

Chemical permanent-wave solutions, hair dyes, hair sprays, cosmetics, deodorants, etc., can clog or damage your skin or hair follicles.

---

**The chemicals can also be absorbed through the skin and cause toxic reactions to your body.**

---

Elizabeth Rose, in her book **Lady of Gray** (1985), has a detailed account about her severe reactions to hair dyes. Nail polish containing chemicals can also make your nails brittle and break easily.

Cooking utensils made of aluminum can have a toxic effect on your body. An increasing volume of research indicates that aluminum from cooking utensils and medications (such as Amphogel) are associated with senile plagues in the brain of the elderly afflicted with Alzheimer's disease.

Dusty furniture or clutter creates a wonderful incubator for yeasts to grow. Old books and newspapers are also covered by yeasts.

*Sophia, a housewife, had been very busy raising four children in a small, crowded apartment. Her priority was driving her children back and forth to different schools. The apartment had been left unkempt and cluttered with piles of old newspapers and magazines. She, her husband and her children suffered from flus and colds all the time, whether there was an epidemic or not.*

A damp environment is also wonderful for yeast overgrowth. Richard is an example.

*After Richard moved to a beachfront apartment, to his surprise, instead of feeling invigorated by the fresh sea breeze, he experienced fatigue, sinus congestion, foggy mind and depression. He noticed that the clothes in his closet and the carpet were damp. There was also mildew under his kitchen sink.*

Soil is another rich ground for yeasts to thrive. Lily had a bad experience after she moved into a garden house.

*Lily was so excited when she moved into a house with large front and back yards. She purchased lots of shrubs to further beautify her gardens. Every time after she dug the soil or worked in the yard, she would suffer from flu-like symptoms such as sneezing, runny nose, headaches, foggy mind and extreme fatigue.*

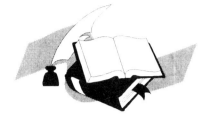

# Chapter 9

# Spiritual Factors

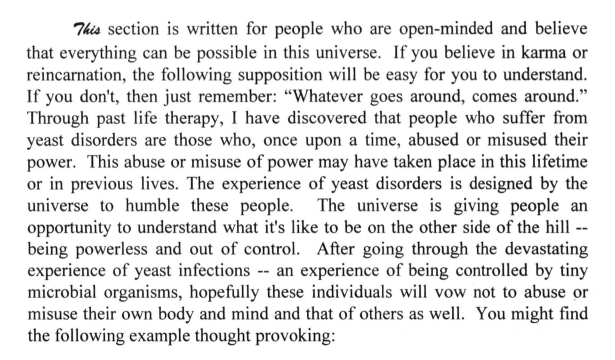

*This* section is written for people who are open-minded and believe that everything can be possible in this universe. If you believe in karma or reincarnation, the following supposition will be easy for you to understand. If you don't, then just remember: "Whatever goes around, comes around." Through past life therapy, I have discovered that people who suffer from yeast disorders are those who, once upon a time, abused or misused their power. This abuse or misuse of power may have taken place in this lifetime or in previous lives. The experience of yeast disorders is designed by the universe to humble these people. The universe is giving people an opportunity to understand what it's like to be on the other side of the hill -- being powerless and out of control. After going through the devastating experience of yeast infections -- an experience of being controlled by tiny microbial organisms, hopefully these individuals will vow not to abuse or misuse their own body and mind and that of others as well. You might find the following example thought provoking:

*Mr. Lee, a 65-year-old Chinese man, immigrated from Taiwan to the United States to join his children after he retired from farming for 40 years. In the early years of his farming in*

*Taiwan, he sprayed some poisonous herbal solution on the vegetable beds once every six months to prevent the bugs from attacking his vegetables. Most of the insects shied away from his vegetable farm because of the unpleasant smell of the poisonous herbal solution. When D.D.T. became available, he took advantage of the convenience and used this chemical pesticide on every single crop. Countless bugs and worms were killed as a result of this frequent spraying of pesticides.*

*After he came to the United States, he kept a very busy life by practicing Tai-Chi every weekend, working in his garden and babysitting for his grandchildren whenever he could. He had become a vegetarian and was content with his new life. However, in the past two years, he had developed a strange sore on his left leg. It came and went. Every time it flared up, it felt like thousands of insects were eating away at his leg. It was red, feverish, and unbearably itchy. After consulting with several physicians, they could not find a clear cause for the infection. Some physicians suggested that he amputate his leg to prevent a possible cancer condition. He decided against the amputation and prayed for forgiveness for his killing of all those insects in the past. In addition, he adopted an anti-yeast diet and Chinese herbs for detoxification. His condition continued to improve.*

# Part IV

# Anti-Yeast Therapy

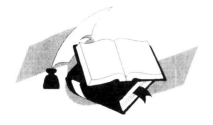

# Chapter 10

# Physical Detoxification and Nourishment

———◆———

*Quick* fixes are commonly sought after by people in contemporary society. Unfortunately, healing takes time. Normally, if a person has been sick for one year, it takes at least one month to heal or recover. Similarly, if a person has been ill for 20 years, then it takes at least 20 months to recover. Knowing this approximate time frame for healing, you need to be patient and committed in order to achieve the best results.

The combination of two or more of the following treatment methods tend to yield better and faster results in physical detoxifying and healing.

## Anti-Yeast Nutritional Program:

The phrase, "anti-yeast nutritional program," instead of anti-yeast diet, is used in this book because the general public tends to think that "diet" denotes reduced calories and boring foods. Anti-yeast nutritional program is nutritious and delicious when your taste buds change for healthy foods. An anti-yeast nutritional program basically consists of no sugar, no dairy, no wheat, no yeast, no alcohol, no caffeine, no nicotine and no chemicals. Most people tend to panic when they hear these "eight commandments." Just remember, habits can be formed and reformed. If you are serious about getting well, then everything can be done! The purpose of an anti-yeast nutritional program is to avoid putting more harmful substances into your body, so that your body will not be taxed all the time.

Sugar, dairy, wheat, yeast, alcohol, caffeine and nicotine products are foods for yeasts. As mentioned previously, when you feed the right foods to yeasts and wrong foods to your body, the yeasts have a great time sucking your nutrition and energy and then deposit toxins in your body. Consequently, you can experience instant fatigue, bloatedness, stomach pain or headache after the ingestion of the favorite foods for yeasts.

### *No Sugar:*

Sugar is poison! Sugar stimulates the thyroid and pancreas to overwork. Continuous overwork of these two vital glands can result in their exhaustion and sluggish metabolic function. Consequently, low energy, hyperactivity, irritability, anxiety, depression, poor mental concentration, and mood swings become common symptoms. Unfortunately, an average American consumes 120 pounds of refined sugar each year! A no sugar diet includes no refined sugar, honey, molasses, maple syrup, corn syrup and concentrated fructose. Melons such as watermelons, honeydews and cantaloupes are high in fructose. Dried fruits such as raisins, apricots and pineapples not only contain a high concentration of fructose, but are loaded with yeasts.

Although strawberries are a favorite fruit for many, they are to be avoided. Some people have severe allergic reactions after eating strawberries. This is not necessarily because of the content of the strawberries, instead, the allergies come from the reactions to yeasts on the surface of strawberries. Have you observed how the strawberries are grown? They sit on the ground or straw all season long until they are picked. The dirt, dust, yeasts and bacterias can stay on the bumpy surface of strawberries and it is difficult to wash them off even if you try. It is also unrealistic to peel the skins when you eat them; therefore, the best way to avoid the reactions is not to eat them, especially when you are actively infected with yeasts.

Grapes are loaded with fructose. Their skins are also covered with yeasts and dust. To prevent rotting, farmers do not wash grapes before they put these appealing fruits in the market. Most people eat grapes without washing or peeling the skin. Even if they do, the high concentration of fructose is also beneficial to yeast growth and detrimental to your health.

Citrus such as oranges and grapefruits are high in fructose and cold in nature (not temperature). Many cultures such as Chinese, Mexican and American Indians are concerned with the hot and cold nature of foods. The Chinese sense of cold and hot is parallel to the concept of yin and yang. Yin denotes characteristics such as cold, depressive, inactive and dark. Yang denotes characteristics such as hot, anxious, active and bright. Because citrus is cold in nature, it depresses the healing process. People who have degenerative diseases or yeast disorders should avoid citrus fruits as should surgery patients.

Apples, pears, bananas and papayas are recommended fruits, but no more than two pieces a day. If constipation is one of your yeast infection symptoms, one apple and one banana a day is usually a good combination to facilitate elimination. If your yeast infection is severe, then peel the skin off the apple and eat the banana when it's just right; don't wait until it becomes too ripe and sugary.

Corn is also loaded with sugar. A little bit of corn sprinkled in your soup or mixed vegetables should not hurt; however, you need to avoid eating a bag of popcorn or a whole corn on the cob if you suffer from severe yeast infections.

If you want to use any sweeteners, brown rice malt or syrup is a good choice. After a digestive process, brown rice malt turns into maltose, which is alkaline in nature. This alkaline can neutralize the acidity in the digestive tract and thus reduce bloatedness and create a comfortable, settled feeling after eating. For years, the Chinese have used rice malt as a remedy for upset stomach. A moderate amount of rice malt is thus recommended for cooking or baking.

### No Dairy:

Dairy products include whole or skim milk, ice cream, cheese, yogurt and butter. These are favorite foods for yeasts and are mucous-producing. Mucous can accumulate in the sinuses, throat, bronchus, lungs and digestive tract. Sinus headaches, sore throats, asthma, bronchial infections, coughs, postnasal drips, halitosis, and constipation are common symptoms associated with mucous problems.

Many people think that milk supplies a rich source of protein and calcium. Protein, yes; calcium, no! Because of the homogenization process, the calcium in milk is difficult for your body to absorb. People who drink a lot of milk end up having calcium deposits in their joints and fingers and developing arthritic symptoms. Some also develop painful kidney stones. Many grains, green leafy vegetables and herbs are rich in absorbable calcium. You should not rely on milk or other dairy products to treat or prevent calcium deficiency.

Drinking a lot of milk to correct calcium deficiency is a myth! Many research studies reveal that when people drink milk to increase calcium intake, they also increase protein intake. When protein intake is high, it produces a high ratio of phosphorus. Phosphorus is acid. In order to balance the Ph of the blood, calcium (an alkaline) is drawn from your bones. This is actually the main cause for osteoporosis (McDougal, 1983; Robbins, 1987).

---

**Many people drink milk or eat dairy products for protein supply. In actuality, your body does not require animal protein. Look at the largest animals in the world such as giraffes, hippopotamuses, elephants, cows and horses; they are vegetarians and they produce their protein through grass, alfalfa, leaves and grains.**

---

An average American, from birth to age 70, eats eight cows, nine pigs and 15,000 eggs. The protein and fat content of a meal often exceeds 50%. According to the American Heart Association guidelines, 20% protein, 20% good fats and 60% complex carbohydrates are safe ranges.

What should you use to substitute for cow's milk then? Soy milk and rice milk which are available in most health food stores are good choices. If you suffer from a severe case of yeast disorder, you may even be allergic to soy. In that case, stick to rice milk first. Later on, when your immune system improves, you may gradually add soy milk to your nutritional plan.

### *No Wheat*:

Wheat gluten is a favorite food for yeasts and is mucous-producing. Most Americans believe that wheat is a nutritious grain and they therefore consume a large amount of wheat products on a daily basis. When you go to a restaurant, the first food item presented to you is usually wheat rolls or crackers. When you go to work or school, you eat wheat bread sandwiches. When you feel like having some carbohydrates, you eat pasta, spaghetti or macaroni. Many of your breakfast cereals also contain wheat. Your favorite pancakes are most likely made of wheat. Wheat is everywhere and it seems to be difficult to avoid.

As a result of consuming a large quantity of wheat, many Americans suffer from sinus congestion, headaches, asthma, and mucus in the respiratory tract. As explained previously, when yeasts are well-fed with their favorite foods such as wheat, they multiply quickly. In addition to sucking your nutrition through their strong, vampire-like hooks, they also deposit toxins after a hearty feast. The toxins they release can cause all kinds of allergy symptoms as described in Chapter 5.

As described in Chapter 2, one of the devastating effects I had experienced before I was able to control yeast disorders was being overweight. For years, I have observed that many Chinese from the northeastern region of mainland China tend to be overweight. A popular portrait of a Shantongese (Shantong is a province in northeastern China) who sells wheat buns in Taiwan is that he has a big belly and a double chin. Chinese from the southern regions of China who live on rice tend to be more slender. This interesting observation has inspired me to stay away from wheat products in addition to the other favorite foods for yeasts. Consequently, I was able to shed 50 pounds of excess weight and to get rid of many devastating yeast disorder symptoms. For more than 25 years, I have been able to maintain my ideal weight and remain free of yeast disorder symptoms!

Brown rice is the least allergy-causing grain on Earth. Brown rice contains useful fiber, protein, complex carbohydrates, vitamins, minerals and an anti-inflammatory substance. Many researchers have begun to use brown rice to treat cancer and AIDS. Brown rice cereals and cakes can be used to substitute wheat cereals and crackers. If you don't have a severe case of yeast disorders, you can also use oat bran muffins, oat bran cereals, oatmeal, and rolled oats for breakfast. If you are allergic to oat products, stick to rice products first. When your health improves, you should be able to add oats to your meals or snacks.

If you are a sandwich eater, you should go to health food stores to look for breads without wheat, sugar, dairy and yeast. This task will be a "treasure-hunt." However, your persistence will eventually pay off.

Pasta, spaghetti and macaroni can be replaced by rice noodles or mung bean (Chinese green beans) noodles. You can find these items in Oriental grocery stores. If you go to a Chinese grocery store, ask for "Me-Fun" (rice noodles) or "Don-Fun" (green bean noodles).

## *No Yeast:*

As mentioned previously, yeasts are everywhere. Yeasts are in the air you breathe, in the water you drink, on the furniture you sit on and in the food you eat. Tap water is often contaminated with yeasts nowadays. After you are used to drinking purified water, you may experience stomachaches when you drink tap water. Leftover foods that you put in the refrigerator may soon become mildewed after a few days.

The most frightening part of all is that yeasts are hidden in most of the *Standard American Diet (SAD)*. Breads, cakes, muffins, bagels, nuts, raw vegetables, surfaces of fruits, soy sauce, and miso soup are loaded with yeasts. Many vitamins also contain yeasts. You can hardly escape the invasion of yeasts if you don't pay special attention to your daily food intake.

Yeasts, no matter what form, can add to the population of the existing yeasts in your body which will exacerbate yeast disorder symptoms. Many women reported that their vaginal yeast disorder flared up after consuming brewer's yeast for a few days. The best way to avoid this devastating effect is to read the labels every time you purchase foods. Avoid ingesting the food items mentioned above.

If you have severe or persistent constipation or diarrhea, you should cook your vegetables. Stir-fried or steamed vegetables are as delicious as raw vegetables (salads) once you change your taste buds. The best way to stir-fry is to use canola or olive oil. These two kinds of oils are mono-unsaturated. Chemically speaking, they have "only one arm sticking out" which means that they have very little chance to be oxidated in the cooking process. Consequently, their nutritional value will not be altered as much by heat as polyunsaturated oil such as safflower oil. Many people favor canola oil because it is odorless and cheaper than olive oil.

Some people believe that raw foods have better nutritional value because they have "life." These people will go to the extreme of avoiding all cooked foods.

> **There are so many nutritional theories out there today that you might feel like you are walking through a jungle. To help you cut through the jungle, I would like to recommend an approach which actually brings satisfactory results to people who are infected with yeasts.**

The fact is that when my clients begin to eat lightly cooked vegetables, their symptoms of constipation, bloatedness or diarrhea improve. Why? The roughness of raw vegetables is very hard for a weak digestive system to handle, which in turn, causes more digestive problems. Furthermore, the surfaces of raw vegetables are loaded with yeasts. Have you ever observed how farmers harvest vegetables? Vegetables are usually sitting in the open air all season long. The dust, dirt, yeast, bacteria and chemical sprays (if not organically grown) stay on the surfaces of the vegetables. Farmers usually don't wash the vegetables when they deliver them to the markets; otherwise, the vegetables would rot easily. Markets don't wash the vegetables before the sale for the same reason. Nowadays many markets spray water periodically on the vegetables to keep them green and looking fresh. That moisture can actually facilitate the growth of yeasts on the vegetables.

Restaurants usually don't wash the vegetables when they fix the salad for you; doing so costs more labor and time. Can you imagine what you are eating when you have a dish of salad? Many people feel instant fatigue or lethargy after they have a big bowl of salad. The reasons are simple: your digestive system is being taxed and the yeast population in your body has instantly increased -- a double whammy! An additional helpful tip is to wash the vegetables very thoroughly before cooking. This will reduce the amount of yeasts which accumulate on the surfaces of the vegetables.

Among the vegetable category, three vegetables should be avoided even if they are cooked. The first are mushrooms. Mushrooms are fungi, members of the yeast family. The second item are tomatoes. Tomatoes are "yin" food. The Chinese concept of cold and hot, or yin and yang, has played a major role in human healing for thousands of years. One of the significant symptoms of yeast disorders is fatigue and low immunity. Because tomatoes are classified as yin food, it would make healing difficult for a fatigued person who has already too much yin chi (sluggish, low energy) to heal. Besides, tomatoes are loaded with natural sodium, which causes water retention. Fluid retention is also a common symptom of yeast disorder. A point worth mentioning is that many hospitals serve tomato juice, sauces or products to patients after surgery. The yin nature and high amount of sodium in tomatoes can hamper the healing process and contribute to wound infections or complications. Nursing mothers should also avoid tomatoes because the yin nature of the food can affect the baby's digestive function and cause diarrhea.

The third item are eggplants. According to the Chinese food/medicine theory, eggplants are not good for kidney functions. Kidneys are heavily responsible for water excretion and circulation. As mentioned previously, water retention is a common symptom of yeast disorders; therefore, it is best to avoid this item in your food consumption.

Nuts, whether raw or roasted, often contain a good amount of yeasts. If you must have nuts, then use almonds. Almonds are considered "king of nuts" because they are easy on the digestive tract, and are rich in protein, fiber, vitamins and cleansing properties according to Chinese medicine and food theories. The best way to enjoy almonds is to purchase raw ones from health food stores. Roast them in the microwave oven for four or five minutes or in the conventional oven for 10 minutes at 400 °F. Set them on the cpunter to cool. Then seal them in a plastic food storage bag and put them in the freezer. Remember, any food should not be stored in the refrigerator for more than three days; otherwise, they mildew. Don't add any salt or oil to the roasted almonds. They are naturally delicious!

The roasting process will kill off the yeast on the surface of almonds. Do not buy almonds which are already roasted. Read the labels -- the roasted almonds or any roasted nuts usually contain added yeasts!

### *No Alcohol*:

Alcohol is a product of fermented wheat, rice and fruits (usually grapes, sometimes other fruits). Fermentation requires yeast. Sugar is a by-product of this fermentation. When drinking alcoholic beverages, you are ingesting yeast, sugar and chemicals all at once -- a triple whammy! Ethanol is a chemical substance which can alter thought processes and clot the liver. Influenced by movies and televisions, the general population believes that alcohol can loosen up a person, which in turn, can contribute to a more romantic lovemaking. Some of my clients reported that they could make love to their partners only after they had a glass of wine or a can of beer. Alcohol beverages can actually cause performance problems in bed. When people stopped drinking socially or habitually, they have found out that "sober sex" is actually far more exciting and enjoyable than "intoxicated sex!" Many men cannot get a satisfactory erection after too many glasses of wine or beer. Ethanol can alter a person's thought processes to the extent that the mind and body do not coordinate or cooperate!

Alcohol is particularly detrimental to a person who is infected with yeasts because of the "triple whammy" effect. Yeasts in the alcohol add to the existing yeast population in the body. Sugar feeds the yeast and thought-altering ethanol can make the foggy mind even foggier!

### *No Caffeine:*

Caffeine is a favorite substance of many Americans. Unfortunately, it is also a favorite food for yeasts. While drinking coffee or tea may be an upper for you, it also makes your little friends in your body, yeasts, very happy! Some people think that they take better care of themselves if they drink decaffeinated beverages. However, even decaffeinated coffee or tea can contain up to three percent of caffeine. A consistent consumption of these decaffeinated beverages can allow caffeine to accumulate in your body, and thus feed the yeasts.

Many people admit that coffee smells good, but doesn't really taste that great when they put it into their mouths. If that is the case with you, why not just smell it, and drink a healthier beverage? Others believe that without coffee, they cannot get going in the morning or cannot carry on during the day. Coffee has become a crutch in their lives. If you review our history, our ancestors seemed to be able to get up early in the morning and work a long day when coffee was not an available item. Habit is formed over time. Fortunately, it can be reformed in a relatively short period of time! Carolyn is a good example:

> *For as long as she could remember, Carolyn had been a caffeine addict. At the time she came to see me for weight management, she drank an average of 30 cups of coffee per day! She was nervous and anxious. Her mental concentration was not as good as it was before. She could not lose weight no matter how she starved herself. Despite all these unfavorable symptoms, Carolyn believed that she must have so many cups of coffee to handle her demanding real estate business and her single parenthood taking care of two young children.*

> *A few weeks into the lifestyle-change program, she reported with great excitement, "I can't believe it! Today I woke up realizing that I haven't had coffee at all for four consecutive days! I am doing just fine with the caffeine-free, cleansing herbal beverage. The funny thing is that I don't even miss coffee. As a matter of fact, I feel more energetic and productive without it! My memory has improved and my hands stopped shaking. Although I suffered a few days of headaches*

*due to caffeine withdrawal, I have no headaches now. What I am most happy with is that I'm losing weight and losing my double chin!"*

### No Nicotine:

Nicotine is another favorite food for yeasts. Even if you are a non-smoker, secondary inhalation can be just as detrimental. A few years ago, I experienced this condition firsthand:

*I had a presentation at an international conference in Madrid, Spain. Almost everyone smoked in Spain. The food was also loaded with sugar, dairy, wheat and yeasts. For two weeks, I was eating ham and cheese sandwiches with hard French bread for lunch almost every day because there were few other choices. To make matters worse, I spoke very little Spanish and to my surprise, the Spanish people spoke even less English! I had lectured in 14 different countries prior to this trip, and I was always able to get by with English. This, of course, added mental stress to my yeast-activated body. Soon I developed a good case of sinus and chest congestion and my voice was hoarse because of the mucous.*

*Many conference attendees suffered the same symptoms and thought they had caught a bad cold. Little did they know that these were typical yeast disorder symptoms mainly caused by the heavy amount of smoke from cigarettes and poor diet. It took me a total of four weeks to recuperate despite the fact that I was symptom-free prior to this trip!*

What happens to people who are smokers? They usually experience excess mucous in their respiratory tracts, raspy or cracking voice, dry and burning eyes, fatigue, bloatedness, and cravings for cigarettes or other favorite foods of yeasts. Yeast overgrowth thus occurs in the body of smokers. This yeast infection can be transmitted to a sexual partner. It can also be transmitted to a baby through the bloodstream and/or birth canal. If a woman smokes during pregnancy, for sure the baby will inherit this infection and manifest it in symptoms such as mid-ear infections, skin rash, colic, sore throats and recurrent flus and colds.

---

**Cigarette smoking is one of the toughest addictions to control. Basically cigarette smoking acts like a pacifier for the smokers. In order to let go of the pacifier, you must find replacements for this "pleasure."**

---

Make an inventory of things which would bring you a lot of pleasure and develop a habit of doing them when you feel like having a cigarette. Delay the cigarette smoking by getting busy with other things which would also bring you pleasure. I had an interesting experience with my daughter in letting go of her pacifier:

*My daughter loved her pacifier when she was an infant. When her teeth began to erupt, I took away her pacifier. She then began to suck her index fingers. First I thought it was kind of a cute behavior and did not discourage her. When she entered preschool, I realized that she had gone too far in this behavior because some of her acquaintances began to tease her. Her index fingers also looked slightly deformed. I was afraid that the shape of her mouth and teeth would also be affected, so I made a deliberate effort to help her stop this addiction.*

*Persuasion did not work. Rubbing Tigerbalm on her index fingers also did not work. She cried as if this was the end of the world, "If you don't let me eat my fingers, what can I eat? I have nothing to eat when I go to bed?" She seemed to have a good point there. I wracked my brain for several days trying to figure out what she could "eat" instead of her index fingers. I did not want to give her food at bedtime for fear that she might develop cavities. Finally I made a list of things she enjoyed most during that time. She loved to give me a "massage" by having me lie on my stomach while she used her little fists to pound on my back. As she did this, I would appear to enjoy her massage very much by sharing a lot of laughter with her.*

*She also liked for me to sing Chinese folk songs and rock her on my lap as I sung to her. Every night I would do these things with her and told her that she did not need to "eat" anything because she would be happy and tired, and she would be able to go to sleep very quickly. Interestingly, she quit her addiction "cold turkey!"*

---

**In addition to using healthy alternatives for pleasure, a combination of psychological counseling to reduce the sense of insecurity, hypnosis for positive reinforcement, Chinese herbal formulas for cleansing toxins, and acupuncture to regenerate the body and cease dependency can work very well in shortening the journey of smoking cessation.**

---

### *No Chemicals*:

Paints, gas stove or car fumes, carpets, hair dyes, tampons, sanitary pads or toilet tissues which contain or are treated by chemical substances can also cause yeast infections. Artificial sweeteners, artificial food coloring and flavoring, drugs (including medication, LSD, heroine, cocaine, marijuana, etc.) are all chemicals. Chemicals can clog the liver and kidneys easily. The liver and kidneys in our bodies are just like an oil filter and a fuel filter in a car. When the oil and fuel filters are clogged, the car can not run smoothly. The same is true with our bodies. When the liver and kidneys are clogged with chemicals, they cannot excrete toxins efficiently. When toxins are backed up, the immune system becomes sluggish. Consequently, the opportunistic organisms such as yeasts are allowed to thrive.

## Herbal Therapy:

For as long as recorded history existed, Chinese and other Asian populations, Egyptians, Africans, Eastern Mediterraneans, South Americans and American Indians have been using herbs to prevent illnesses and to treat ailments. Industrialization and modernization have influenced some parts of the world to move toward western medicine and away from herbal remedies. In a fast-paced society, people tend to go for the quick fix. When people experience headaches, instead of getting more rest or relaxation, or taking herbs which may be brain nourishing, they often reach for the aspirin bottle or other pain killers. If the headache is not too severe, within 30 minutes they may see the results. After people develop the "aspirin mentality," they tend to treat all illnesses the same way.

Unfortunately, most western drugs only inhibit the inflammation or disease process; they do not treat the core problems to heal the body. However, because most Americans have no time to wait, they tend to go for drug (chemical) treatment over and over again until their bodies collapse or diseases worsen. They actually waste more time, money and energy in the long run!

---

**Yeast disorder is not something drugs can treat, because drugs are a major cause for the disease to begin with. Besides, as mentioned earlier, yeast has 250,000 to 350,000 species; no single drug can kill them all!**

---

## Which Herbs Are Good for You?

Basically, there are three categories of herbs: poisonous, medicinal and food-grade herbs. Poisonous herbs are used to combat life-threatening diseases such as cancer or severe allergies. In the old days, when the body became poisonous, an experienced Chinese herbologist would use poisonous herbs to get rid of poisons in the body quickly. Poisonous herbs can kill if the dosage is not carefully monitored. Because malpractice lawsuits are quite fashionable in our contemporary society, even a very experienced herbologist of our day will shy away from poisonous herbs to avoid the risks.

Nowadays, medicinal herbs are used popularly in both Asian countries and the United States. A prolonged use of medicinal herbs can cause side effects just like western drugs. For example, long-term use of goldenseal root or dandelion can cause effects similar to antibiotics. Excessive use of white willow bark can cause stomach lining irritation much like aspirin.

Food-grade herbs are the herbs used by the Chinese and other people as food on a regular basis. For example, many eldery Chinese grow herbs in their back yards. When these herbs mature, they pick the leaves and/or stems and stir-fry them with other vegetables or make herbal soups with them. My mother prepares herbal dishes on a regular basis for better lung capacity, eyesight, blood circulation, energy flow and so on.

### *How Do the Herbs Work?*

The state of art of using food-grade herbs is the formulation. Single herbs usually are not as effective as combined herbs. When herbs are properly formulated, one herb will take care of the other herb's side effects and enhance each other's main effects. Several pointers regarding formulation are worth mentioning. First, the quality of herbs determines the potency of the formulation. When the herbal ingredients are healthy and strong, the formula will have greater effectiveness. That's why you will see great variations in the prices of herbs. For example, the price for one pound of ginseng can range from $20 to $400.

Second, when the quantity of each herbal ingredient in a formula changes, the effectiveness of that formula also changes. For example, a formula containing one portion of A, two portions of B and three portions of C, versus a formula containing one portion of C, two portions of B and three portions of A, can be quite different in its potency and effectiveness. Therefore, a bottle of herbal formula listing the same ingredients as another brand, does not mean that the two brands have exactly the same effects.

The final point is that during the formulation process, the amount of water and heat used, and the way the formula is prepared, also makes a difference in its potency and effectiveness. For the above reasons, going to a health food store to pick up a bottle of "good" herbs could be like searching for a needle in a haystack. It is advisable to consult with experienced health practitioners who are knowledgeable about herbal formulations.

In the old days, people usually had to go to Chinatown to see an herbologist to get a dash of this, a pinch of that, and finally a total of 10 to 20 kinds of herbs in one pouch. They went home with perhaps 21 pouches for a week's supply and had to boil each pouch of herbs in four to eight cups of water until the water was reduced to one small cup. By that time, the whole house smelled. Worst of all, they had to pinch their noses, lock their eyebrows and swallow the bitter potion three times a day for at least one week. Luckily, those days are gone! Most herbal formulas are available in clean, easy-to-take capsule form.

Some of you may wonder why herbal capsules are much larger than typical western drugs? The reason is simple. Western drugs are usually highly processed and condensed. Because of this, western drugs are usually very potent and deliver many side effects. As mentioned previously, one herbal formula can contain as many as 10 to 20 ingredients, so it is difficult to condense into a small capsule. Even though some of you may have to practice swallowing them, the benefits of doing so will certainly outweigh the inconvenience.

> **How do food-grade herbal formulas work?** Basically, they **nourish your body cells and certain organs and glands. When a body is in an unhealthy state, the cells look like wrinkled, unhappy faces because they are dehydrated and loaded with toxins. Food-grade herbs act like a summer rainfall to a dry and cracked rice field -- your malnourished body.**

When the drought is over, the rice field becomes fertile ground for a healthy crop. By the same token, when your body is well nourished by these herbal concentrates, your body cells will resemble a smiling, full moon. They are happy and full of vigor. In this state your immune system will be strong and able to defend your body against invasions from yeasts, bacteria, viruses, parasites and other foreign agents.

### *Are There Any Side Effects?*

Well-formulated herbs do not have side effects. However, they might have cleansing effects called "cleansing crisis." The major functions of herbal formulas are detoxifying and healing. Since toxins take many years to accumulate, they also take time to cleanse. During the cleansing process, you may feel worse before you feel better! If you have a severe case of yeast disorders, in the first few days of the herbal therapy, you usually feel better because your malnourished body quickly soaks in the nutrients in the formula.

For a while your body cells may be half asleep because of dehydration, malnourishment and invasion of toxic substances. When they are nourished, they begin to wake up and have the ability to look around and see who does not belong there! Pretty soon they spot the toxins and begin to push them out of the cells. When these toxins are purged out of your body cells, they get into the bloodstream and circulate throughout the body. This is the time when you will feel "very sick." Another reason for feeling "sick" at this time is the *yeast-die-off syndrome*. When you begin to feed your body with the right foods and starve the yeasts, their vampire-like hooks begin to weaken and finally fall off the mucous membranes of your body. As mentioned previously, they "drop dead" or "commit suicide!"

> **Right before yeasts die, like any other beings, they will struggle for survival by screaming out, "Feed me! Feed me!" This is the time you may feel a tremendous craving for yeast-favorite foods such as sugar, dairy, wheat, and yeast products. If you give in, you lose the battle! After giving in, they will be strong again and continue to haunt you.**

In addition to cravings, the cleansing symptoms may include headaches, sinus congestion, runny nose, sore throat, bronchial congestion, abdominal pain, bloatedness and general malaise. These symptoms resemble flus and colds; thus, many people tend to rush to their "regular doctor" (M.D.) to get some antibiotics to "kill" the infection. When these symptoms are inhibited by antibiotics, they temporarily feel better and believe that they have received the right treatment.   Unfortunately, the vicious cycle will continue to repeat until they gain insight into what is really going on.

> **When cleansing symptoms occur, just feel great about feeling miserable!  You actually have two choices at this time.  The first is to tough it out and allow the cleansing to take place faster so that you can get better sooner.  The second choice is that you reduce the dosage of the herbal formulas that you are taking; therefore, the cleansing effects will not be so vigorous.  This will reduce your discomfort, but will also slow down the healing process.**

Some of the clients that I have dealt with deliberately took a few days off from work to go through the cleansing crisis.   The choice is yours because it's your body with which you are dealing!   The following interesting, yet sad example will help you understand this concept better:

*Janet has been a vegetarian for more than 10 years and believed that her body was quite clean. Unfortunately, her face broke out after being exposed to some sheets in a hotel which might have been laundered with chemicals.   Since then she began to search for a cure.   When she came to my office, she began to recognize that it was not just the sheets in the hotel that caused her skin to break out; it was also because of her diet.   Her diet contained many foods that supported the growth of yeasts.*

*A few days after she started the anti-yeast nutritional program and herbal therapy, she began to feel better. However, starting from the second week her face looked worse. Large pimples erupted all over her face.   Even though she was cautioned about the cleansing crisis, she panicked and rushed herself to a "famous" dermatologist in Beverly Hills.   The dermatologist injected cortisone into a few of the largest pimples on the left side of her face to make them shrink.*

*The cortisone shrunk these pimples so effectively that it created several deep recessions on the left side of her face. By contrast, the smaller pimples on the right side of her face which she left alone, healed beautifully after the cleansing crisis. When she attended one of my seminars, she showed the audience both sides of her face to demonstrate the difference between western medicine and alternative medicine!*

### Why Herbs?

Why herbs? Many people claim that since they eat very healthfully, they don't need any supplements such as herbs or vitamins. Theoretically they are correct, but in practice they are not. Vegetables or fruits are usually picked by farmers before they are mature. Otherwise, they can spoil easily. This is a very logical and economical thing for the farmers to do. However, after eating "premature" produce day in and day out, consumers can become malnourished. Worse yet, the chemical sprays and fertilizers in the produce can also clog your liver and suppress your immune system.

Food-grade herbs provide concentrated nutrition. Since they usually come in a highly concentrated form, they can work fast to cleanse and nourish the body. Even if you grow your own produce in your back yard and pick them fresh and ripe everyday, the air you breathe and the physical and psychological environments you are exposed to can still cause you nutritional deficiencies.

### Would I Get Addicted to Herbs?

Some people are concerned about getting "addicted" to food-grade herbs. Since these herbs are foods, they can be eaten just like any healthy food items such as carrots, broccoli or celery. Are you afraid of getting addicted to carrots or broccoli? If the answer is no, the same can be applied to food-grade herbs. Even if you are "addicted" to these herbs, the "side effects" would be too much energy or eliminating a lot of waste. If that's the case, don't you think that these are the kind of "side effects" you desire?

*Where Do I Get Good Quality Herbs?*

Generally speaking, it is safer to consult with health professionals who are experienced in dispensing herbs. Many brands of herbal formulas are available in health food stores nowadays. Usually their prices are lower than those dispensed by health professionals. However, many of my clients reported that the results of herbal formulas they obtained from health food stores were usually not as good as those from health professionals. As mentioned previously, the quality of herbs, formulation and preparation procedure are major factors in determining the effectiveness of a formula. An experienced and conscientious health professional is usually familiar with the different application of each formula. You may pay a little more for the herbal formulas obtained from a health professional; however, you could also shorten your journey of trial and error. You may save money in the long run.

An additional benefit for consulting with a health professional is that when you go through the cleansing crisis, the experienced professional can monitor the progress or guide you through the process effectively. The professional advice and support you will get from an experienced health professional usually will outweigh the few dollars you save at health food stores.

## Exercise:

As you are aware, exercise improves blood circulation and increases energy flow. Many people complain that they feel exhausted after a long day's work. They just want to collapse on the sofa or bed and go into a coma! Interestingly, once they push themselves to go out to do light exercise, or better yet, slow walking, they feel energized afterwards. As mentioned previously, lack of exercise can cause sluggish blood flow. A stagnant environment can become an incubator for yeasts to overgrow. When blood circulation is smooth, toxins in the body can also be flushed out more easily.

Many people believe that the only way they can exercise is to go to the gym. In order to go to the gym, they have to purchase a membership, set a certain schedule and bring the exercise outfit with them to work. All this of course is "extra work" for people who are busy and in most cases, lazy! Therefore, they would create the excuse that they are not "ready" to exercise yet.

> **Prior to the availability of gyms, how did our ancestors exercise? They just walked or got involved in physical activities such as household chores or outdoor chores. Simplicity is beauty. Why not adopt the most simple form of exercise: walking?**

One hour of walking can reduce 300 calories. Slow walking is the preferred form of exercise for people who are not used to vigorous exercise or people who don't have a whole lot of energy. Depending on your energy level, you may start from 10 minutes of slow walking to 30 minutes or one hour a day. Choose the best time of the day you can walk consistently. Some people prefer to do it before or after work, while others walk during their lunch break. If you can choose a location where there are trees and/or flowers with white clouds and blue skies, the effect will be further enhanced. If not, walking around in a shopping mall is just fine.

When you walk, don't think! Most people think too much! Their minds have constant traffic which are often worse than the Ventura Freeway or San Diego Freeway in southern California. Allow your mind to unwind. Just enjoy the trees, flowers and birds and sing with the universe. If you really cannot help thinking, then talk to God or your higher self. Say something like this:

*"Thank you God (or the universe) for giving me such a beautiful day! Thank you for helping me get on the right track. Now I need your further assistance to make more progress. Please give me strength, courage, resources and guidance to stay on the right track to improve my health (business, relationships, etc.)."*

Or, you can say an affirmation like this one:

*"I now enjoy great health, energy and happiness."*

Repeat these kind of statements 300 times a day and visualize the desired results as you say these affirmations. You will see dramatic results after 21 days!

Slow walking is for everybody and is *free of charge* -- you don't have to pay membership fees! It is also safe for all ages, sexes and races. If you walk constantly every day, you will see tremendous positive results on your cardiovascular, digestive, respiratory and nervous systems. Some of my clients reported that they felt a natural sense of happiness while they slow walked. Guess what?

> **Slow walking helps release endorphins which can give you a high, but calm feeling. It's like you are on drugs without the ill effects! Once you develop a routine to do slow walking, you will be "addicted" to it. This is one of the best addictions you could ever have in life!**

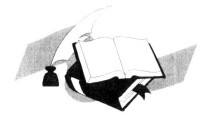

# Chapter 11

# Psychological Detoxification and Nourishment

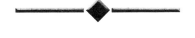

**When** people suffer a severe case of yeast disorders, not only are their bodies toxic, but so are their minds! These people usually have had traumatic childhood or early adulthood experiences which have made them angry, resentful, frustrated, regretful and negative. As mentioned previously, carrying negative emotions day in and day out is just like driving your car with the hand brake on. It will cause a lot of wear and tear on your immune system! *Based on my experiences counseling thousands of people thus far, I have found that psychological stress is actually the most important cause for adult onset of yeast disorders! If these negative emotions are not released effectively, the rest of the regimens discussed so far would only provide a temporary relief.*

It is like cleaning up a vast field of tall weeds. An anti-yeast nutritional program, herbal therapy, exercise and other treatment methods only serve the function of chopping down the weeds above the ground. Psychological detoxification and nourishment serve to uproot the core problem from underground. If this uprooting is not done, the field may appear to be clean for a while. Nevertheless, when the summer rainfall comes, the weeds will grow like crazy again. Similarly, when a person is confronted with some life crisis, the problem of yeast disorders may reoccur! Psychotherapy, meditation and hypnosis are some useful ways to combat this.

## Psychotherapy:

Many theories have been employed in psychotherapy. Some of the most commonly used include: Sigmund Freud's psychoanalysis, Edmund Husserl's existential analysis, Alfred Adler's individual psychology, Carl Roger's client-centered therapy, Harry Stack Sullivan's interpersonal relations theory, Albert Ellis' rational emotive therapy, B. F. Skinner's behavior modification, Frederick (Fritz) Perls' Gestalt therapy, Eric Berne's transactional analysis (Corsini, 1979), Virginia Satir's conjoint family therapy (Satir, 1967) and Irvin Yalom's group psychotherapy (Yalom, 1979). The list goes on.

> **Experienced psychotherapists usually combine several theoretical frameworks instead of being based on just one theory, for no theory is complete. When therapists can pull together the theories they have learned in school and their own life experiences, and come up with their own styles, this is the time they can be most effective.**

When I taught psychotherapy theory courses at the University of California, Los Angeles to the graduate students in the Psychiatric/Mental Health Nursing program, I used to tell them my favorite little story:

*A little monk went to a famous temple to see a Master to learn kung fu. The Master taught him ten approaches and sent him home to practice. When the little monk returned as instructed, the Master asked him, "How many approaches do you remember?"*

*The little monk replied, "Eight."*

*The Master said, "Good! Go home and continue practicing."*

*When the little monk returned the second time, the master asked again, "How many approaches do you remember?"*

*The little monk replied with some degree of embarrassment, "Five."*

*The Master said, "Good! Go home and practice some more!"*

*When the little monk returned the third time, the Master again asked the same question. He replied with greater embarrassment, "Three."*

*The Master responded with joy, "My little brother, you are doing great!"*

*The little monk was puzzled, so he asked the Master for an explanation. The Master said, "Brother, when someday you remember only one approach, that one will be your own. At that time I will retire and have you take over my temple!"*

---

**Whatever theories your therapist uses is not important. The important thing is whether he or she can help you work through the emotional issues which have been haunting you for years. The most common emotional issues usually come from intergenerational relationships. Many people harbor anger, resentment, guilt, regret or fear because they have not resolved certain emotional issues with their parents.**

---

The following case example will shed some light on this.

*Gretta, a 34-year-old woman, was on disability when she came to me for help. She stated that she had been very healthy and energetic all her life up until the last two or three years. She suffered from a severe case of allergies, chronic fatigue, poor mental concentration, lower back pain, neck and shoulder strain and depression. She had seen numerous holistic health practitioners in the past two years without any obvious improvement. In addition to putting her on the anti-yeast nutritional program and Chinese herbal therapy, I also worked with her vigorously on her emotional conflicts with her mother.*

*According to her, her mother was once a very bright and successful business woman. For some reason her mother managed to lose her business and everything she owned and became homeless. She would disappear for months and Gretta would not have the faintest idea where to locate her. This had been going on for more than five years and had driven Gretta crazy. Her anger, resentment, frustration, shame and guilt was mounting despite the fact that she was a very spiritual person and had tried many ways and means to release her negative feelings toward her mother.*

*Through a spiritual psychotherapy process, Gretta gradually understood why she was challenged with this situation. With guidance, she wrote a very frank letter to her mother recounting all the positive and negative aspects of the interactions between her and her mother and asked for mutual understanding, acceptance, forgiveness and release. In the course of writing this letter (about four months), Gretta went through a process of psychological cleansing which I call "psychological diarrhea." She revisited the frustration, anguish, and disappointment she had had since childhood. After the letter was revised and polished to perfection, I asked her to burn it since we did not know where her mother was at that time.*

*A couple of months later her mother reappeared in her life and offered to babysit for her young daughter and newborn baby. She was able to accept the offer since most of her "psychological toxins" had been purged when she finished the letter. They continued to work through many issues and Gretta's yeast disorder symptoms also continued to dissipate. Eight months after she started the treatment, she was able to resume a full-time position at work looking and feeling healthy and happy!*

The key in the psychotherapeutic process is to release any negative emotions that have accumulated over time. *You may believe that you have already forgiven whomever has done you wrong, whether it be your spouse, parents, children, siblings, relatives, partners, friends, or co-workers. However, if you still suffer from any physical or mental ailment, that is an indication that you may have chopped off the tops of the weeds but have not dug out the roots.*

Writing a spiritual letter as mentioned above is a very effective way to release the deep emotions which you may not be aware of on the conscious level. *This letter is very powerful for it can be very constructive or destructive. Never share this letter with anyone until it has been revised and polished with proper guidance from an experienced therapist.* This letter can be written to persons living or deceased. This is because people (including spirits -- if you believe in them!) are connected by energy, and energy can travel through the universe freely if it's strong enough! The following is the format for this powerful letter.

### First Paragraph:

Start with positive remarks about the person you are writing the letter to. If you have been carrying a great deal of anger and resentment toward this person, this paragraph will be very difficult for you to write. However, it is essential for you to spend time to recollect all positive memories about this person. Pretend that you are the recipient of this letter; wouldn't you like the letter to begin with positive remarks instead of negative ones? Substantiate every statement you make with specific scenarios.

### Second Paragraph:

After you pour out all the positive remarks about the person, move on to the negative ones. This "however" section should be easy for you if you have been very angry and resentful. In the first draft of the letter you can say whatever you want. If you have to swear, feel free to do so! This is your chance to let it all out. Remember, do not share the early drafts of this letter with just anyone! The "psychological diarrhea" you experience in this stage is to be shared with your experienced therapist only! During the time that you are writing this paragraph, be warned that you may experience increasing anger, resentment and sadness. If you need to cry a whole lake of tears, do so!  If you need to yell and scream, go ahead!  Just do it when you are alone and remember to close the doors and windows so your neighbors will not think that you are crazy.  You may also tear the letter into pieces and start all over again if this will help release some of your anger.

---

**Whatever you do at this stage, make sure that you don't hurt yourself or others.  The purpose is to release, not to hurt!**

---

### *Third Paragraph:*

In this paragraph you bring everything together in a positive and sensible manner.  You state that the purpose of this letter is not to badger nor blame; instead, it is intended to help the person understand how his or her behavior has affected yours.  State that you would like to hear a sincere apology from the person, and that you offer your apology as well for any of your behavior which may have upset the person.  Remember, if the recipient of the letter is around at the moment,  he or she may also have a lot to say about your behavior.  The mutual apology and forgiveness will lead to mutual acceptance and release so that you can move on with your new life!

The following is an example of a letter using the principles explained above:

*Dear Mother,*

*I remember you used to dress me nicely and take me to school.  The dresses you made for me had drawn a lot of attention to me and admiration from my teachers and classmates.  You were also a very good baker.  All the cookies, cakes and pies were wonderful treats for me when you were not drinking.  You were very friendly with people and well liked. You worked so hard to provide me and my brothers with a comfortable material life.  I want to let you know that I appreciate all this very much, although I did not express my appreciation often in the past.  These positive attributes have influenced my behavior and have contributed to a comfortable material life for me today.*

*However, my heart aches everytime I remember the harsh words you used to criticize me. You used to call me "stupid" or "lazy." No matter how hard I tried, I was not good enough for you. Since I was six years old, I helped you take care of my two little brothers while you worked nights in a hospital. I remember one morning when you got home from work, you criticized me for not putting my brothers to bed on time the previous night and not covering them with enough blankets. I felt that you treated me like a maid. When my brothers and I were all in school, you scolded me for not helping my brothers do their homework. When you were drinking, many times I had to cancel my party plans with my classmates for fear that they would see you drunk. When you had verbal and physical fights with father, my legs were trembling and I was so scared that you might kill each other. All these negative incidences have influenced my life in a very negative way. Today, I have an addictive personality just like you did. My addiction is food, instead of alcohol. I frequently stuff myself with the same kind of cookies, cakes and pies that you used to bake for me when I am lonely and depressed. Those kinds of foods mean love to me even though I know they make my body bloat up and make my mind foggy. I have trouble finishing many projects I've started. I cannot express my feelings effectively or sometimes I just don't feel anything. As a result, I am having trouble with my marriage and children. I know I am critical to my husband and children. I often catch myself using the same language you used to criticize them. "Stupid" or "lazy" are just some examples. Since I don't have love and respect for myself, it is hard for me to love and respect others, including my family.*

*The purpose of this letter is not to blame or badger you. I know you had a rough life losing your mother to cancer at age three and later battling your husband's inability to support the family. It seems to me that all your life you felt alone because you did not get the support and love you needed and wanted. I just want to let you know how your behavior has affected mine in both positive and negative ways. **For the positive part, I want to express my sincere appreciation. For the negative*** *part, I would like to hear a sincere apology from you! I also apologize for any of my behavior which might have upset you. We both did not upset each other on purpose, because we simply did not know better! I forgive you for being an imperfect mother. Please also forgive me for being an imperfect daughter! With this mutual apology and forgiveness, I hope we can release each other so that we can move on with our lives. I hope you receive this letter with an open mind and a loving heart!*

*Unconditional love and peace,*

*Deborah*

---

**As demonstrated above, the four major steps in the psychological healing process involve *understanding, acceptance, forgiveness and release (letting go).* When these four steps are accomplished, basically you are home free! If any of these four steps are incomplete, then you will manifest dysfunctional behavior.**

---

Dysfunctional behavior is the kind of behavior that jeopardizes the quality of your life, including your health and happiness. Dysfunctional behavior was, at one time, survival behavior. For example, if you grew up in a family where your parent(s) had drinking problems, you might have to develop behavior such as no talking, no feeling and no trusting. Your drinking parents' behavior could have been very unstable and unpredictable. One moment they might be very loving and giving, but the next moment they could be very violent and abusive. This unpredictability may have made you develop the tendency not to talk, to feel nor to trust so that you would not set yourself up for disappointment nor punishment.

This type of behavior may have helped you survive difficult times during childhood and enabled you to move on. However, during adulthood, this kind of behavior can sabotage your relationships with romantic partners, spouses, children and co-workers. The best way to correct this behavior is to go through the process of **understanding** why your parents had drinking problems, **accepting** the way your parents were (are), **forgiving** your parents for robbing you of a happy childhood, and **letting go** of your anger and resentment. Unfortunately, many people *prefer* to carry grudges because their parents had done them wrong and they feel their anger and resentment is well justified. What they don't realize is that they are actually hurting themselves more than anyone else. Although it is difficult to be positive and forgiving in the beginning, with practice, it can become easier and easier. Comparatively speaking, it actually takes more energy to stay angry and negative. Consider the following Zen Buddhist story:

> *Two monks were travelling on foot. When they reached the bank of the river, they saw a woman who was trying to cross the river. After rainfall, the usually shallow river had filled with rapid running water. It was getting dark and the young woman was hesitant to cross that seemingly dangerous river. One of the monks volunteered to carry her on his back and in such a manner safely reached the other side of the riverbank. He let her off his back, said goodbye and hurried on.*
>
> *The two monks rested at a deserted temple that night. The monk who carried the woman across the river was quickly sound asleep. The other monk, however, was tossing back and forth. Finally he shook the shoulder of the sleeping monk. The awakened monk said, "Brother, what's the matter? Why are you still awake? Come on, get some sleep. We have a long journey tomorrow!"*
>
> *The other monk answered angrily, "How can you sleep after what you have done today? We are monks. We are not supposed to look women straight in the eye. How dare you carry a young woman over your shoulders and think nothing of it? How dare you?!"*
>
> *Here was the reply: "Brother, when I reached the riverbank, I dropped the woman off my back. Why do you still carry her over your shoulders?"*

Dysfunctional behavior served a purpose at one point, but now it's time to let go, and move on! Otherwise, consider the consequences.

Negative emotions not only rob you of a peaceful life, they are also linked with degenerative diseases such as AIDS, cancer, Chronic Fatigue Syndrome, Crohn's disease, lupus, multiple sclerosis, and yeast disorders. Don't you prefer to live more comfortably?

## Meditation:

Meditation is a practice to achieve a state of calmness and peace. Some people also use this practice to train the mind to develop insight. When the mind is centered, the body functions better. Many people report that both their mental and physical health improve after a period of meditation. There are many theories or schools you may use for meditation. Taking a meditation class from an experienced teacher or guru is a good way to learn how to meditate effectively.

In the western world, people are always pressured for time. There is fast food, fast photo, and so on. Thus, I came up with "fast meditation" to suit the needs of people in a contemporary society! Based on my more than twenty years of experience in meditation, I have designed a 10-minute meditation which can quickly help you quiet your mind and give you a sense of peace and deep relaxation.

> **There are 1,440 minutes in a day. If you cannot spare 10 minutes to do this "fast meditation," you are not serious in improving the quality of your life!**

You can do this "fast meditation" almost any time. Just don't do it while you are driving. Otherwise, you may end up on the wrong side of the road! Some people do it in the morning; some in the afternoon; others, in the evening. Whatever schedule you can work out is fine. The key is that you be consistent. Like everything else, practice makes perfect! The following is the procedure:

1.  Wear comfortable clothing. If you do this during a break at work, undo your tie or belt, take off your eyeglasses, and kick off your shoes.

2.  Sit on the floor with your back supported by the wall, or sit in bed with your back supported by the headboard. Keep the spinal column straight but not overextended. Your legs are crossed and folded. The lotus posture gives you the best results if you can do it. If you cannot fold your legs comfortably, just fold them anyway you want, as long as you can sit still for 10 minutes or more.

3.  Draw your chin inward toward the neck.

4.  Put your tongue in its natural place.

5.  Relax your shoulders and allow your lungs to expand well.

6.  Keep your eyes half open and fixed on a point about one foot from your feet. If you find this difficult, just close your eyes.

7.  Begin deep breathing. Breathe in through your nose and breathe out through your mouth. When you breathe in, imagine you are inhaling fresh and warm air, clean energy, and peace. When you breathe out, you are exhaling heavy and cold air, fatigue energy and tension. When you breathe in, close your mouth; when you breathe out, open your mouth. While exhaling, it's as if you are blowing air into a balloon very gently.

8.  After you get used to the deep breathing, coordinate your breathing with relaxation. Breathe in slowly, and let go the tension in your feet while you breathe out. With every breath, you continue to release the tension in your legs, then knees, thighs, hips, lower abdomen, stomach, chest, back, hands, shoulders, neck, face and forehead. Remember to start from the feet and move upward to your head.

9.  As you breathe in and out and release the tension from toe to head, your entire body will begin to relax. Continue deep breathing and allow your body to feel very light -- so light, that there is no boundary between your body and the room in which you are sitting. Continue the deep breathing, and you will feel that there is no boundary between your body and the universe. At this point, you may have an out-of-body experience. Don't dwell on that experience. Just return to a normal

pattern of breathing -- breathe in and out through your nose as you normally do.

10. Now, nothing is on your mind. Your mind is now empty, blank. It's so quiet, so peaceful. Nothing is on your mind. You are now in a deep state of relaxation. So quiet and peaceful. You may stay in this deep state of relaxation for as long as you want to. When you are ready, you just count: one, two, three, then open your eyes and bring yourself back to the awakened state. You then can get up and go ahead to do whatever you want to do and feel good about it!

If you are very uptight and one round of a 10-minute meditation cannot calm you down, just repeat the process again. You can repeat this process as many times as necessary to unwind your mind and achieve that heavenly state of peace. Some people have found that an instructional tape is very helpful, especially when they are too tired to concentrate on the total process. You may order these tapes using the order form at the end of this book. All the meditation or hypnosis tapes I have made contain no music. This is because some people find that music can be distracting. If you prefer, you may incorporate your favorite music into our meditation tape or procedure.

This 10-minute fast meditation has dramatic effects on relaxing your mind and body. If you do this two or three times a day on a daily basis, you will experience marked improvement in mental clarity, blood circulation, and general well-being.

## Self-Hypnosis:

The term "hypnosis" comes from the Greek root "hypnos," meaning sleep. According to Spielgel (1972), hypnosis is an altered state of awareness in which the individual withdraws his peripheral awareness and concentrates all attention on a focused goal. Thus, hypnosis is a state somewhere between sleep and wakefulness, an altered state of consciousness that occurs in a continuum of awareness. When attention has been keenly focused, there may be amnesia or lack of memory. This is a trance state. The trance state, often synonymous with the hypnotic state, is characterized by a modified sensorium and an altered psychological state (Zahourek,

1985). In a therapeutic trance state, according to Milton Erickson, "the limits of one's usual frame of reference and beliefs are temporarily altered, so one can be receptive to other patterns of association and modes of mental functioning that are more conducive to problem solving" (Erickson & Rossi, 1979, p. 3).

The early roots of hypnosis can be found in the ancient writings of the Egyptians, Chinese and Hindus, where rhythmic chanting and drumming were often followed by a semi-sleep state. In this state, individuals would perform unusual physiological endurance, such as walking across hot coals or lying on a bed of nails. It is Franz Anton Mesmer (1734-1815), however, who is credited with being the founding father of hypnosis, although the term hypnosis was not used until much later. Mesmer believed that the planets influenced humans via a magnetic force, which was responsible for the state of human health. By redirecting the magnetic flow, one can restore health and energy.

In 1843, James Braid (1795-1860), a Scottish surgeon, coined the term "hypnosis" in his publication "Rationale of Nervous Sleep." He is an important historical figure because he asserted that no special power or force passed from the operator to the subject; rather, it was the unusual suggestibility of the subject to the operator that resulted in hypnotic states. In other words, all hypnosis is self-hypnosis!

Self-hypnosis theories and techniques were further developed and refined by John Elliotson, a prominent English physician; James Esdaile, a Scottish surgeon; Jean Marie Charcott, a French neurologist; and Sigmund Freud, a renowned neurologist. Although proven successful as a form of surgical anesthesia and an aid to health problems, hypnosis was not popularly utilized until World War II. During World War II, hypnosis was used in conjunction with traditional analytic approaches to combat "battle fatigue" or "battlefield neurosis." During the Korean War, hypnosis was also used for mind control and "brainwashing" (Larkin, 1985). In the late 1960's and early 1970's, public interest in alternative approaches to mental and physical health refueled interest in the study of hypnosis.

Taking note of the above history, it is clear that hypnosis has come a long way! Today, hypnosis is not only used for anesthesia, it is used for pain management, addiction control, goal attainment, and health enhancement as well. In the case of severe yeast disorders, hypnosis (or self-hypnosis) can be used to ingest powerful, positive thoughts into the subconscious mind to induce healing. It can also be used to uncover and discharge negative emotions of which you may or may not be aware. In other words, self-hypnosis can be applied, in conjunction with other treatment modalities, to enhance both physical and mental health. Both are much needed in the course of treatment for yeast disorders.

When I use self-hypnosis to facilitate the healing process for people with yeast disorders, I usually make an individualized tape based on that person's particular symptoms and needs. The tape is made while the client is in my office. The client then takes the tape home and listens to the tape at least once a day. The most susceptible time is bedtime. An autostop tape recorder is preferred because it does not require one to get up and turn off the tape when it is done. *Basically, the client sleeps with powerful suggestions pounding into their subconscious mind. When the original symptoms improve, a new tape can be made with a new set of suggestions.*

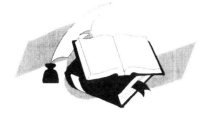

# Chapter 12

# Environmental Cleansing

———◆———

*As* discussed earlier, yeasts are everywhere! Wipe your furniture regularly to avoid the accumulation of dust and yeast. Clean the areas under your kitchen and bathroom sinks. Make sure that your gas stove is functioning well and without leakage. Keep your carpet dry and clean, or live in a home with hardwood floors. Clean your refrigerator frequently. Scrub your bathtub and shower stall regularly to avoid mildew. Chop down the trees and shrubs in your yard if you are allergic to the pollen. Use an air freshener at home or in the office to keep the air clean. Avoid using chemical substances such as hair dyes. Stay away from a newly painted room. Wear a mask when you clean up your garage or work in the yard.

Avoid using permanent solutions, hair dyes, hair sprays, shampoos and conditioners containing chemicals. Some beauty salons are beginning to use natural substances for hair care. Many health food stores also carry natural personal care products such as deodorant, shampoos, conditioners and soap. Keep your nails clean, well-trimmed and free of chemical nail polish.

Use cooking utensils which are made of stainless steel, glass, ceramic, wood or bamboo. Avoid using aluminum or iron utensils. Avoid using mercury to fill your cavities. Heavy metals can clog your liver and kidneys and lower your immune function. This, in turn, can cause heavy metal poisoning.

**The general idea is to keep your environment as clean, yeast-free and heavy metal-free as possible. When necessary and feasible, you may want to consider moving to an area where the air is dry and clean. All these may not cure your yeast disorders, but will certainly control the amount of yeasts in your environment and reduce the severity of the problem.**

# Chapter 13

# Spiritual Cleansing

———◆———

*As* mentioned previously, this section is written for people who are open-minded and believe that anything is possible in the universe. If you believe that the universal energy is a powerful resource at your disposal, this chapter will offer you very useful guidance in terms of how you can activate it to help you achieve your goals within the least possible time (Tien, 1996). This chapter will address two important aspects: first, how to release negative energy and bring about a positive outcome within the least possible time; second, how current life situations (or suffering) can be related to previous life experiences and how they can be improved or corrected. Our discussion here is of course based on the belief that there are lives after lives. For those of you who don't believe in reincarnation, just read this section as entertaining pieces of information. Ruminate on this information from time to time, and perhaps someday you will develop a new understanding and belief.

## Releasing Negative Energy:

The following is an extremely powerful technique for releasing negative emotions or feelings about any person or situation. *Use it only for positive purposes.* The initial steps (1 through 9) are basically the same as those described in the meditation procedure in Chapter 11. Starting from Step 10, is another set of techniques for "blowing up" negative energy or bringing about positive outcomes.

> **The reason why this technique can be used for dual purposes is that you are sending a strong message to the universe, and asking the universe to bring you results, whether releasing negative energy or generating positve energy. Once you send your message to the universe, don't worry about how things are going to work out. Let the universe (God) work out the details and bring you nice surprises!**

To make it easier for you to follow, I will repeat the first nine steps.

1. Wear comfortable clothing. If you do this during a break at work, undo your tie or belt, take off your eyeglasses, and kick off your shoes.

2. Sit on the floor with your back supported by the wall, or sit in bed with your back supported by the headboard. Keep the spinal column straight but not overextended. Your legs are crossed and folded. The lotus posture gives you the best results if you can do it. If you cannot fold your legs comfortably, just fold them anyway you want, as long as you can sit still for 10 minutes or more.

3. Draw your chin inward toward the neck.

4. Put your tongue in its natural place.

5. Relax your shoulders and allow your lungs to expand well.

6. Keep your eyes half open and fixed on a point about one foot from your feet. If you find this difficult to do, just close your eyes.

7. Begin deep breathing. Breathe in through your nose and breathe out through your mouth. When you breathe in, imagine you are inhaling fresh and warm air, clean energy, and peace. When you breathe out, you are exhaling heavy and cold air, fatigue energy and tension. When you breathe in, close your mouth; when you breathe out, open your mouth. While exhaling, it's as if you are blowing air into a balloon very gently.

8. After you get used to the deep breathing, coordinate your breathing with relaxation. Breathe in slowly, and let go of the tension in your feet while you breathe out. With every breath, you continue to release the tension in your legs, then knees, thighs, hips, lower abdomen, stomach, chest, back, hands, shoulders, neck, face and forehead. Remember to start from the feet upward to your head.

9. As you breathe in and out and release the tension from toe to head, your entire body will begin to relax. Continue deep breathing and allow your body to feel very light; so light, that there is no boundary between your body and the room in which you are sitting. Continue deep breathing, and you will feel that there is no boundary between your body and the universe. At this point, you may have an out-of-body experience. Don't dwell on that experience. Just return your breathing to its normal pattern: breathe in and out through your nose as you normally do.

10. Now, imagine there is a central point between your two hip bones (or between the two ovaries for females). This is your first chakra. Mentally see that there is a golden rope wrapping around your first chakra. The rope then goes all the way down through the chair to the center of the earth. At the center of the earth there is a golden post. The other end of this golden rope is now wrapping around the post. You are now "grounded" and connected with the earth energy, an important part of the universal energy.

11. Mentally see that there is a point of light between your temples called theseventh chakra. "Turn on" the light and envision that your head is illuminated with golden light.

12. Say hello to yourself silently and hear your voice return the greeting. If you hear someone else's voice, tell that person to leave. This is a sacred place reserved for you only.

13. Mentally see your entire body surrounded by a ring of oval-shaped golden light. This light is about 18-inches thick. You are now protected by this golden light.

14. If you are troubled by an event or person, mentally see that there is a rose in front of you (outside the golden light). This rose can be of any color you like. Say, you are concerned about your health; put that worrisome energy in the rose.

15. Ignite a stick of imaginary dynamite in the rose and "blow up" the rose loaded with your worries. As the whole thing blows up, it turns into golden dust. This golden dust is now showering over your head and your entire body, and reinforcing your existing golden light and positive energy. You can repeat this part as many times as you want. You can "blow up" a whole garden of roses with the negative energy you want to release, or with the positive outcome you want to bring about. For example, if you wish to have a nice house, just put the image of that house in the rose and blow it up with the rose. You can also use this technique to blow up your health concerns such as pain or depression, or concerns about your relationships. *Remember, only blow up the energy of a person or a situation. Do not blow up the person you don't like. If you are too angry to follow this guideline, wait until you are calmer. This technique can only be used for a positive intent. Otherwise, you might have to take the consequences for the misuse of this technique.*

---

**This procedure can release the negative energy which is hovering over you. After practicing this technique frequently, you may be surprised by the miraculous solutions which the universe may bring to you. Basically, you just release your concerns of any nature to the universe and trust that the solutions will come at the right time in a perfect way!**

## Past-Life Therapy:

In 1981 a Gallup poll revealed that 38 million Americans now believe that they have had past lives -- about one-fourth of the adult population (Talbot, 1987). In my 28 years of practice, I have been surprised and delighted to find that more and more intelligent and educated people from all walks of life believe in reincarnation or at least keep an open mind about it. In Britain, polls by the conservative *Sunday Telegraph* showed that belief in reincarnation by the general public had risen from 18 to 28 percent in a 10-year period (Woolger, 1988). This growing interest in reincarnation is not limited to the general public. Increasing numbers of psychotherapists and medical doctors are using past-life regression techniques to help their clients overcome physical and psychological health problems (Weiss, 1988). Psychotherapists and hypnotherapists like Morris Netherton in California and Joe Scranton in England have demonstrated on film and television their fascinating work involving past-life regression in adults.

In Jungian psychology, Carl Gustav Jung, the Swiss psychologist and psychiatrist, asserted that the place where all psychotherapy must begin is in the "personal unconscious" (Jung, 1973). As a great synthesizer and visionary of the 20th century, Jung offered a broad bridge allowing the differing traffic of psychology, religion, literature and science to pass over and do productive business with each other (Woolger, 1988). The emphases on self-examination, dream analysis, visualization and imagery in Jungian training have paved a path for many psychotherapists to deepen their interest in research in past-life regression techniques.

In my therapeutic work, I combine traditional psychotherapy and past- life regression techniques. Therefore, *I prefer to refer to the process as past-life therapy, instead of past-life regression.* Woolger (1988, p. 13) in his book, **Other Lives, Other Selves** has made the point very clear: "Past-life exploration can be like taking the lid off Pandora's Box; it can unleash potent forces over which we may have little control. For this reason, it is my firm belief that guiding regressions and research into past lives should only be undertaken by those fully trained in psychotherapy."

In the case of yeast disorders, a cluster of symptoms are often present (see Chapter 5). However, each individual can have different kinds of ailments. Each symptom, whether it is physical or psychological in nature, may be related to a different type of past-life experience. June's case is a good example.

> *June, an attractive, intelligent, 32-year-old woman, came to me with symptoms of chronic fatigue, allergies, bloatedness and eating disorders. She also suffered from depression and low self-esteem because she was out of a job. When she experienced spurts of emotional eating, she often stuffed herself with favorite foods containing sugar, dairy, wheat and yeast. During those binging episodes, she ate so fast and so much that her jaws and stomach hurt. After she was put on the anti-yeast nutritional program, she would still binge on healthy food from time to time. Portion-control was a serious problem for her. Knowing that she believed in reincarnation and that she had been meditating, I suggested past-life therapy be used as a technique to release some of her deep emotional issues. She was thrilled to try it.*

> *After a deep breathing and induction procedure, the following was revealed: June "saw" herself as an old, female beggar in England during the 14th century. Most of her life she was starved. One time, there was a festival in the countryside. She sneaked into the crowd and stuffed food into her mouth as fast as she could for two reasons: she had been starved and she was afraid that people might ask her to leave as soon as they spotted her. She ate so fast that her jaws and her stomach hurt.*

> *Through reprogramming, June was able to let go of the traumatic experience associated with food and allow positive images to stay with her. In the process of reprogramming, I suggested that she "see" herself formally invited to the festival and eating slowly with grace and moderation. She enjoyed the food and the event. She also enjoyed the abundance of resources. A few weeks after this past-life therapy session, she reported that she found a new job that was something she liked doing and also paid well. Also, her eating habits dramatically improved.*

*To account for her low self-esteem or not loving herself, a few more past life therapy sessions were rendered. She "saw" the following scene: A little girl was drawing an apple at a table. After she finished drawing, she colored the big apple purple. She liked it so much that she proudly showed it to her dad. To her surprise, her father shouted at her, "What in the world are you doing? Why did you color the apple purple? I have never seen a purple apple in my life!" His tone was that of ridicule. Tears were streaming down June's little face, but her father never noticed.*

*As a grown-up, although highly intelligent and competent, June did not think much of herself. She was always very hard on herself. She would criticize herself harshly before anyone else had a chance. This, of course, was rooted in her father's being critical and non-supportive of her. During reprogramming, I suggested that she "see" a different picture when she presented a purple apple to her father.*

*Instead of ridiculing her, her father greeted her with a big smile and compliment, "What a beautiful apple! Purple! I've never seen such a beautiful apple in my life! You are so creative, my darling!" June proudly smiled and continued to draw more purple apples....*

---

**As you can see, past-life therapy is not only used to deal with traumatic experiences in previous lives, it is also used to reprogram unpleasant experiences in this lifetime. Whatever might come up during a therapy session, depends on what is significant to you subconsciously. The past-life therapist simply acts as a chauffeur. The chauffeur's job is to ensure that you have a safe ride, but you are the one who decides where you want to go.**

---

In order to have a "smooth ride," I have found that the following preparations are helpful.

**Step 1. Physical cleansing:**

When possible, stay on the anti-yeast nutritional program (see Chapter 10) for at least one month. The anti-yeast nutritional program as described previously will control yeast overgrowth and thus prevent you from accumulating more toxins. Chinese herbal therapy (see Chapter 10) is also important for cleansing the pre-existing toxins in the body. When toxins in your body are minimized, your mind will be better able to concentrate.

Most importantly, clear your body of all alcohol and drugs. Any alcoholic beverages or stimulants such as marijuana, LSD, cocaine, etc., can alter your thought processes and make it difficult for you to concentrate and tap into your subconscious mind for hidden information. If you are on heavy prescription medication, you need to consider alternatives such as herbal remedies to control your disease processes first. When you can taper off your medication to the greatest possible extent, your liver will be cleaner and your mind will be clearer.

Regular exercises such as walking or moderate jogging can improve your blood circulation and increase mental clarity. Tai chi and yoga can also be excellent exercises to relax your body and improve your mental concentration. If you suffer from a severe case of yeast disorders, vigorous exercise can exhaust your body which can in turn cause fatigue and an inability to concentrate. Start from gentle exercises and slowly build up.

**Step 2. Meditation:**

The ability to concentrate can be trained. The meditation technique described in Chapter 11 is a good start for beginners. Meditation is a highly effective method for emptying your mind and relaxing your body. When your mind is as busy as the San Diego Freeway or Ventura Freeway in southern California, naturally it is difficult for you to concentrate. During the meditation process, when you breathe in and out deeply, slowly and steadily, you set the pace for your entire physical and emotional system. This pace will allow you to enter a deep state of relaxation. When your mind is empty and uncluttered, that's the time you can uncover the wealth of information stored in the subconscious.

## Step 3. Self-permission:

Many people are skeptical about past-life therapy because they are not sure that they believe in reincarnation. An interesting phenomenon I have found after thousands of past-life therapy sessions with my clients, is that whether you believe in it or not, it works!

Past life therapy is, by far, the most powerful therapeutic technique available to mankind to release deep emotional traumas. If you just give yourself permission to get well, and give it a sincere try, then you will see results.

> **Many of my clients felt like they had just seen a bad movie when they came out of their trance. However, the mere fact that they were able to revisit the traumatic experience usually gave them a sense of relief. The relief came from the realization that no matter how traumatic their past experiences were, they still had a chance to come back to another life and start all over again! In other words, no matter how bad things might have seemed, it was not the end of the world!**

Another benefit experienced by my clients is the reprogramming that I orchestrated during past-life therapy sessions. The reprogramming, as illustrated earlier, gives clients a new set of positive thoughts to work with. It is not unusual that after a few sessions of past-life therapy, clients experience major breakthroughs such as finding a new job they like, encountering an ideal mate, getting rid of tough physical ailments, and so forth. *The bottom line is that past-life therapy is designed for people to get well, not to prove whether there is reincarnation or not. Therefore, if you give yourself permission to make a positive change in your life, then you will be able to get into your subconscious mind for guidance and solutions!*

Theoretically, everyone can be regressed and is able to "see" what needs to be revealed. However, over the years, I have found that some people have more difficulty than others in benefiting from past-life therapy. For example, people with AIDS have often taken heavy dosages of medication such as AZT and antibiotics. For fear of their lives, they usually don't want to discontinue or reduce the dosage of the drugs they are taking. This, in turn, makes it very difficult to have a clean physical system and clear mind. Similarly, drug addicts and alcoholics have more trouble than others getting into the trance-like state necessary for a successful past-life therapy session.

Another category of people who might have difficulty with past-life therapy are those who have a tremendous fear of revisiting their traumatic past life experiences. Holocaust, torture, starvation, being killed in a war, or being beheaded, hanged or burned to death are but a few examples of these experiences. Again, only when they give themselves permission to "see" what needs to be seen, may past-life therapy provide them with insight and the wisdom to move forward in the present life.

# Part V

# Alternative Treatment Methods

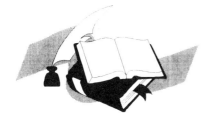

# Chapter 14

# Acupuncture and Moxibustion

———◆———

*Physical*, psychological, environmental and spiritual cleansing basically provide you with guidance to change your lifestyle or certain habits that are not functional. Change is necessary for growth. However, not everyone is ready for a drastic change. Most people are comfortable with the status quo. For that reason, the chapters that follow are recommendations of treatment methods which allow you to rely on health professionals to initiate the healing process. For those who are resistant to change, these treatment methods may serve as a temporary bridge to a greater degree of healing.

## Acupuncture:

For thousands of years, the Chinese have been using acupuncture and moxibustion to regenerate the body and to treat ailments. **The Internal Classic**, written during the Warring States Period (484-221 B.C.), makes up 70 to 80 percent of the current coverage on acupuncture and moxibustion. *A Classic of Acupuncture and Moxibustion* and *The Illustrated Chart of Acupoints and Therapeutic Importance of Acupuncture and Moxibustion* compiled by Huang Fumi (215-282 A.D.) during the Jin Dynasty is regarded as an authoritative monograph in China and the world. Following the publication of this classic, a number of famous acupuncturists of different dynasties continued to make brilliant contributions to the development of acupuncture and moxibustion. They include: Sun Simia (581-682 A.D.) during the Tang Dynasty, Wang Weiyi (987-1067 A.D.) during the Song Dynasty, Hua Boren during the Yuan Dynasty (in the 14th century), and Gao Wu and Yang Jizhou during the Ming Dynasty (in the 16th century) (Chen & Deng, 1989).

After the establishment of the People's Republic of China, the field of acupuncture and moxibustion was rejuvenated because of the government's policy on developing traditional Chinese medicine. In Taiwan, some universities have also incorporated both western medicine and traditional Chinese medicine in their curricula for medical students. The normalization of the political relationship between the United States and China initiated by former President Nixon opened a door for acupuncture to be introduced to America. Since then, acupuncture has gradually established itself in the health care arena of the western world. Today, many health insurance policies provide coverage for acupuncture as a viable treatment modality for many ailments, especially pain management.

In acupuncture, very thin gold, silver or stainless steel needles are inserted into exactly determined points on the skin (acupoints), which are sensitive to pressure. This procedure is designed for therapeutic and/or diagnostic purposes when treating functional, reversible illnesses. Acupoints are like junctions of crossroads. When these acupoints are stimulated by the needles, the body begins to release natural chemical substances called endorphins. Endorphins are "morphine from within." They work like morphine, a painkiller. That's why people can experience almost instant pain relief after receiving the acupuncture treatment. In addition to pain relief, endorphins also give people a high, but calm feeling.

*In the case of severe yeast disorders, the individual usually has an array of symptoms from head to toe. For each symptom, different acupoints can be used to stimulate energy flow, and thus, facilitate the cleansing and healing process.* For example, if the symptoms of low energy and fatigue are present, then acupoints for regenerating the liver, pancreas, thyroid and kidneys will be used. Similarly, if the symptoms of constipation or diarrhea, bloatedness, ulcer, colitis, etc., are present, then acupoints for revitalizing the digestive tract will be used. An experienced acupuncturist will be able to make the best judgment in terms of which acupoints should be stimulated and for how long.

Another purpose of acupuncture is to restore the yin and yang balance. The term yin-yang first appeared in ***The Book of Changes*** (Cheng, 1990). Yin and yang are philosophical polarities, like light and dark, warm and cold, day and night, man and woman, etc. Yin and yang reflect all the forms and characteristics existing in the universe. They act simultaneously in the body and are antagonists at the same time. Complete balance of these two forces maintains perfect health. Thus, they can be compared somewhat with the terms sympathetic and parasympathetic, or adrenergic and cholinergic. These two forces are components of life energy. Maintaining this energy and producing the best possible balance of yin and yang is the dominating element of ancient Chinese medicine (Bischko, 1978).

## Moxibustion:

Moxibustion treats and prevents diseases through application of heat to acupoints or certain locations on the body. Moxibustion and acupuncture have been combined in clinical practice; thus, they are usually termed together in Chinese medicine. When a disease fails to respond to medication and acupuncture, moxibustion is usually suggested. In moxibustion, the leaves of artemisia vulgaris, which is a species of chrysanthemum, are used. They are called "moxa-wool" and usually come in the form of a cone or stick. The moxa leaf is bitter and acrid, producing warmth when used in small amounts and strong heat when used in large amounts. It is of pure yang nature, having the ability to restore yang chi (chi means energy flow or life force). According to Cheng (1990), it can open the twelve regular meridians, travel through the three yin meridians to regulate blood circulation, expel cold sensations and dampness, warm the uterus, stop bleeding, warm the spleen and stomach, regulate menstruation and ease the fetus.

In the case of severe yeast disorders, the yin and yang balance is off. Through the stimulation of certain master and symptomatic points, acupuncture can work wonders for the balancing and healing process.

Moxibustion can also be used to restore yang chi for those who suffer from fatigue and sluggish metabolism. Unfortunately, many Americans often dislike the smell produced by the artemisia vulgaris leaves and choose not to use moxibustion in the course of their treatment.

Nowadays, because of the AIDS scare, most acupuncturists use disposable needles. For those of you who are afraid of needles, the best way to overcome it is to try it. Initially, just try a few needles, then gradually increases usage when you feel more comfortable. Many people associate acupuncture with injections seen in hospitals. Injections require hollow needles which puncture' the blood vessels, thus causing bleeding. As mentioned previously, acupuncture uses very thin, solid, stainless needles. When these needles are inserted, they "slip" between vessels instead of puncturing them. That's why you usually don't see blood after the treatment is done.

---

**Many people who were initially afraid of needles got used to acupuncture after they tried the "graduated exposure" approach. In fact, they grew to like it because of the dramatic results they got from the treatment.**

---

# Chapter 15

# Chiropractic

———◆———

*Chiropractic* has a relatively shorter history than acupuncture. However, it has quickly become a common treatment modality for pain management and other ailments in the past few decades. The first reportedly successful application of chiropractic was in a small town in Iowa on September 18, 1895. A self-educated healer named Daniel David Palmer cured janitor Harvey Lillard's deafness by manipulating his spine back into alignment. Palmer became the first chiropractor. He was also the first in a long line to be imprisoned for practicing medicine without a license!

D. D. Palmer believed that cause and cure for all *dis-ease* was inside the body. Out of his characteristically uninhibited thinking and living patterns, came a new form of uninhibited thinking: the discovery of vertebral subluxation as the cause of all *dis-ease*; and a method of correction by hand only. Although D. D. Palmer did not rediscover the concept of "nnate" from the Greeks, he was the pioneer in drawing the concept of "innate intelligence" from the mental vacuum and pounding it into the consciousness of men.

D. D. Palmer's family, including his son, Bartlett Joshua Palmer; his daughter-in-law, Mable Heath Palmer; and his grandson, David D. Palmer, had helped develop chiropractic into a profession (Mayard, 1977). Although most states were licensing chiropractors by the late 1950s, the medical society's prejudice and hostility continued for years. Starting in the early 1970s a number of studies concluded that spinal manipulation in the hands of an educated chiropractor was safe and effective in relieving musculoskeletal symptoms such as back pain and migraine headaches.

> **Chiropractic adjustment is designed to remove the nervous interference caused by misaligned vertebrae. The removal of nervous interference helps relieve aches and pains. Furthermore, it turns on the healing power of the body. It allows the body's innate intelligence to facilitate energy flow and increase the general well-being of the body.**

Consequently, the individual who receives chiropractic adjustment may also experience relief of allergy symptoms such as hay fever, asthma, chronic fatigue, constipation and sleep disorders which are often associated with yeast disorders.

Since our bodies often experience subluxation knowingly or unknowingly, it is a good idea to have chiropractic adjustments periodically. Just like you visit your dentists regularly to ensure your dental health, you want to visit a chiropractor regularly to ensure your spinal alignment. Don't wait until you have a severe case of yeast disorders to visit a chiropractor!

Nowadays, different chiropractors may use different adjustment techniques. Diversified, craniosacral, kinesiology, Directional-Non-Force Technique (DNFT) and network are but a few examples. You may want to try out different approaches and find out with which one you feel most comfortable.

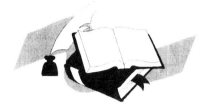

# Chapter 16

# Hands-On Healing

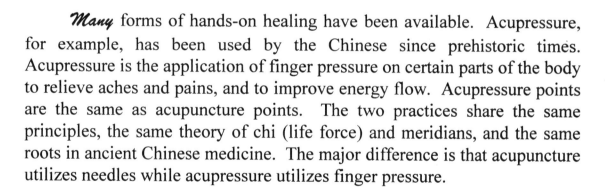

*Many* forms of hands-on healing have been available. Acupressure, for example, has been used by the Chinese since prehistoric times. Acupressure is the application of finger pressure on certain parts of the body to relieve aches and pains, and to improve energy flow. Acupressure points are the same as acupuncture points. The two practices share the same principles, the same theory of chi (life force) and meridians, and the same roots in ancient Chinese medicine. The major difference is that acupuncture utilizes needles while acupressure utilizes finger pressure.

Although acupressure does not yield the same effect as acupuncture in terms of the intensity of stimulation and speed of recovery, if you use it constantly, you will still see marked results in the improvement of symptoms of aches and pains, stress, menstrual cramps, arthritis, asthma, flus and colds, digestive problems and energy level. When coupled with other treatment modalities, acupressure can shorten the healing journey for yeast disorders. If you are into self-healing, taking a class for acupressure will give you a lifelong ticket to better health and higher energy.

Other forms of hands-on healing practices such as massage therapy, therapeutic touch, applied kinesiology, Rolfing, Alexander technique, Hellerwork, reflexology and Jin-Shin Do can also be helpful in the healing process. Massage therapy alone has many schools. Chinese Tui-Na, Japanese Shiatsu, Swedish massage and deep tissue (muscle) massage are but a few commonly known schools (Feltman,1989). Many massage therapists have developed their own techniques. The basic principles of all hands-on healing techniques are the same: facilitating energy flow and improving general well-being.

---

**In case you are confused about which one to choose, here is the simple principle: if it helps you feel better, continue; if you don't feel any difference after you have received the treatment for a while, then why bother?**

---

If your budget permits, try out different hands-on healing techniques to determine which one works best for your health conditions. ***Many roads lead to Rome.*** As long as you get results, that's what counts!

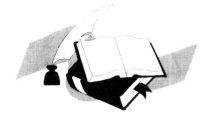

# Chapter 17

# Biofeedback

———◆———

*Biofeedback* is a procedure using physiological amplifiers and filters to accurately record and process biological signals, and feed them back to individuals in a form that is easily comprehended. The field of applied biofeedback began in the United States in the late 1950s. It is the result of a convergence of many separate disciplines including visceral learning theory, psychophysiology, behavioral therapy, relaxation techniques, stress management, biomedical engineering, single motor unit control, electromyography (EMG), and electroencephalographic (EEG) feedback.

The major purpose of biofeedback is to increase your awareness so that your mind has the ability to control your physiological reactivity. Through this awareness, you are able to consciously regulate your physical reactions to stress with the help of biofeedback equipment. When your physical reactions are regulated (namely, your physical relaxation is induced), then mind relaxation will follow (Schwartz and Associates, 1987).

Biofeedback is known to be effective in treating physical illnesses and managing psychological stress. Tension headaches, stomach ulcers, incontinence, bed-wetting, essential hypertension, neuromuscular re-education, anxiety and Attention Deficit Disorder (ADD) are but a few examples.

When you suffer from a severe case of yeast disorders, you usually have a history of chronic stress. Psychological stress can cause wear and tear on the body, and thus cause tension, fatigue and headaches.

> **Biofeedback is a viable method to reduce both physical and psychological tension. When a state of relaxation is accomplished, you will have a better ability to handle more stress and to recuperate physically.**

# Part VI

# Yeast-Related Health Problems

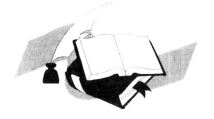

# Chapter 18

# Overweight Problems

◆

*Excess* weight is a very costly health problem which can be associated with life threatening conditions such as atherosclerosis, hypertension, diabetes, cancer, respiratory disorders, gallbladder disease and metabolic dysfunction. Being overweight can negatively affect health, appearance, self-esteem, and even earning potential. Some researchers estimate that each pound of extra fat can cost an executive $1,000 a year in income.

## Causes of Overweight Problems:

Major causes of being overweight include poor eating habits, yeast disorders, thyroid dysfunction, psychological stress and spiritual imbalance.

## *Poor Eating Habits:*

As mentioned previously, an average American eats 120 pounds of sugar per year. From birth to age 70, on the average, an American eats eight cows, nine pigs and 15,000 eggs. A well-balanced diet should contain less than 20% fat, less than 20% protein and more than 40% complex carbohydrates. Excess intake of fat, protein and sugar can turn into overstorage of fat. Americans also tend to overeat or not to eat at regular hours. Some skip breakfasts and others have big meals right before bedtime. Irregular hours and portions can confuse your biological clock and jeopardize your metabolic function.

## *Yeast Disorders:*

As described in previous chapters, yeast disorders are misdiagnosed and improperly treated by most medical professionals. In addition to all the symptoms mentioned in Chapter 5, a persistent overweight condition can be an indication that your metabolic function is being jeopardized by stubborn yeast disorders. Yeast can creep in to any part of your body, especially sites which are weak to begin with. For instance, if your thyroid gland is weak, then opportunistic yeasts can particularly affect your metabolic function and cause further deterioration. If yeast disorders are not corrected, the weight problem will persist. Some clients complained to me that they gained weight even if they just drank water! Even though they may not have been as innocent as they portrayed themselves to be, there is some degree of reality in their complaint. The fact is that it is very difficult for them to lose weight, no matter how hard they try.

## *Hypothyroidism:*

Severe hypothyroidism manifests symptoms such as obesity, constipation, dry skin, cold intolerance, hair loss, puffy face and mental retardation. Contributing factors include congenital and environmental causes. The latter includes poor eating habits. Constant excessive consumption of sugar causes overwork and exhaustion of the thyroid gland. On top of it all, untreated yeast disorders will further weaken thyroid function.

## *Psychological Stress:*

Some people manage to be in constant crises. For those who are used to a dysfunctional behavioral pattern, they feel anxious or uneasy if their lives are peaceful. Somehow they have to create a situation where there will be chaos, and thus their frantic behavior can be justified.

> **People who are not able to manage stress effectively will usually indulge themselves in emotional eating. Food is a symbol of love and comfort across cultures, especially for those who associate food with parental approval and attention.**

## *Spiritual Imbalance:*

Many overweight people suffer from spiritual imbalance because they carry a great deal of "unfinished business" on their shoulders. In most cases, they crave approval from their parents. Some are angry and hurt because they were abused sexually, mentally or physically during their childhood. The predominant emotions are anger, resentment, grief and regret. Some even feel sorry for themselves and feel that their negative feelings are well justified. Usually they are unclear about the purpose of their existences. They tend to "live to eat," instead of "eat to live."

## Treatment for Overweight Conditions:

In order to correct weight problems, you need to learn to nourish your body and mind on a regular basis. Getting and staying trim is a lifelong project. No crash diets, injections, medications, or surgeries can achieve this purpose.

### *Anti-Yeast Nutritional Program:*

The first step toward the right direction is to wean yourself from foods containing sugar, dairy, wheat, yeast, alcohol, caffeine, nicotine and chemicals (Tien-Hyatt, 1990). Stop putting poisonous or highly allergic foods into your body. Give your thyroid a chance to rest and regenerate. Allow your body to avoid the assault of wrong foods, and be nourished by nutrients from the right kind of foods. Review Chapter 10 of this book, and learn what to eat and what not to eat from *Healthy and Tasty: Anti-Yeast Cooking* (Tien, 1997).

### *Herbal Therapy:*

For those of you who have a long history of being overweight, you need to consider herbal formulas specifically designed for weight control as an additional measure. An anti-yeast nutritional program is for giving your body a new start; while an herbal program is for eliminating the existing toxins in your body and revitalizing your sluggish metabolism. A well-formulated herbal program for weight control should have the following three functions:

## 1. Control Your Appetite:

Most Americans overeat. When I travelled in Europe, I noticed that my American friends were often surprised by the relatively smaller portions of food they got in European restaurants. A traditional Chinese belief is that you should not eat more than a handful of food for each meal. For those of you who love to eat, you probably wish that you had a larger hand now (smile)! Even though some of you are well aware of what you should eat and what you shouldn't eat, when an abundance of food is available, your will power often gives in. Luckily, a well-put-together herbal formula can curb your appetite naturally without your trying hard!

## 2. Eliminate Fats from Foods:

As mentioned previously, the Standard American Diet (SAD) usually contains 40% to 60% fat in a given meal (A cheesburger is a good example.) If you wish to reduce weight, you need to learn to eat sensibly and avoid foods containing a high amount of fat. However, as a human being, sometimes you deviate knowingly or unknowingly. A good herbal formula for weight control will also eliminate a good portion of the fat you put in your body. In other words, before the newly ingested fats have a chance to be stored in your body, these herbal formulas will be able to expel them provided that you are not overloading your body with fatty foods all the time.

## 3. Burn the Existing Fat in Your Body and Turn It into Energy:

In addition to preventing new fats from getting into or being stored in your body, the third function of an effective herbal weight control formula is to burn the existing fat in your system and turn it into useful energy. As a result, you will feel energetic, mentally clear and productive.

As described previously in Chapter 10, you might go through a period of cleansing crisis if you have a lot of toxins accumulated in your system. Before your body can function at its optimal level, it has to clean house! Drink a lot of water or caffeine-free herbal tea to flush the debris; therefore, the cleansing and purging processes can be facilitated.

## *Manage Your Stress Effectively:*

Psychological stress, if managed properly, can be motivating and beneficial. The first step is to accept instead of resist stress. Accept the fact that you are being challenged and that every challenge gives you an opportunity to grow and expand.

---

**Life is like school: before you can obtain a diploma or degree, you must be willing and able to do your homework and pass a series of tests, whether you like it or not. The good news is that even if you fail, the universe will provide you with unlimited opportunities to go through the tests again and again until you past them! Therefore, your clock is not ticking. *Time is irrelevant!***

---

Follow the instructions in Chapter 11 to release your *psychological toxins* and allow yourself to move on with your life with a clean slate. If psychological stress becomes paralyzing, then you should seek competent professional help. Hypnotherapy, meditation, acupuncture, acupressure, chiropractic, massage, biofeedback, exercise and an anti-yeast nutritional approach can also be helpful in reducing stress physically and psychologically.

## *Restore Spiritual Balance:*

Spiritually speaking, we all chose our destiny when we were born into this life. No matter what kind of life situation we are in, we are given an opportunity to prove that we have the strength, tenacity, wisdom and faith to overcome obstacles and excel.

> **The only way to get out of the rut of a dysfunctional life situation is to exercise your unconditional love and wisdom.**

Use the principles described in Chapter 11 to understand, accept, forgive and release. Once you can release the negative emotions toward those who have done you wrong, you can release the negative past that has been haunting you. *When you no longer carry the old baggage, you no longer carry the excess weight!* Love and respect yourself as the most unique, creative and miraculous person in the world. If you cannot accomplish this on your own, seeking help from a spiritually-oriented, well-grounded therapist can be fruitful.

Your weight and health problems did not occur overnight. Naturally, becoming trim and getting well takes time. Only your understanding of the illness and wellness process, commitment and patience will bring you positive and permanent results!

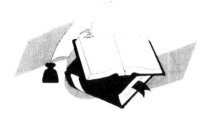

# Chapter 19

# Underweight Problems

◆

*If* you happen to be underweight, you may be envied by a lot of people. They see you as a "lucky minority." If those envious people only knew that you suffer from persistent fatigue, headaches, foggy mind, muscle aches, and alternate diarrhea and constipation, then they probably would not like to be in your shoes!

## Causes of Underweight Problems:

An increasing number of Americans are suffering from underweight problems. This condition is often associated with infections caused by yeasts, parasites, bacteria or viruses. The above microbial organisms usually come hand-in-hand like good sisters and brothers.

## Yeast Infections:

As detailed in Chapters 6 through 9, yeast infections can be caused by physical, psychological, environmental or spiritual factors.

> **Once yeast overgrowth occurs in your body, your cells and tissues will be fermented. This fermentation process makes your cells and tissues lose their ability to absorb nutrients to nourish your body. A phenomenon of "wasting away" is thus present.**

When your body cells are fermented, they also lose the ability to defend you against invaders such as parasites, bacteria and viruses. In fact, the fermentation process will create an environment for parasites, bacteria and viruses to develop a colony and have great parties one after another!

## Parasitic Infections:

We like to believe that developed countries have no sanitation problems. However, the meat, fish and vegetables we eat and the tap water we drink often carry yeasts and parasites. A common parasitic infection affecting many Americans today is giardia lamblia. This has become the number one cause of waterborne disease in the United States. Tapeworms from beef, and baiantidium and trichna (very tiny worms) from pork are also causing infections in human intestines.

Hulda Clark (1993), after years of research on parasitic infections, reported that parasites are responsible for many human ailments. For example, eczema is due to roundworms; seizures, schizophrenia and depression are caused by a roundworm called ascarid getting into the brain; asthma is caused by ascarid in the lungs; diabetes is caused by the pancreatic fluke (a flatworm) of cattle, eurytrema; migraine headaches are caused by the threadworm, strongyloides; acne is caused by leshmania;

heart disease is cause by dog worm, dirofilaria; cancer is caused by a flatworm, the fluke; and the list goes on.    Dr. Clark stressed that in the parasitic infection cases she studied,   all of them (100%) have propyl alcohol in their bodies.  In other words, in order for parasites to be present, your body cells have to be fermented by yeasts first!  Without that fermented environment, parasites will not be able to survive, because your normal cells have the ability to kill these invaders before they have a chance to complete their life cycles.

---

**As you can see, yeasts and parasites have a symbiotic relationship like Siamese twins!  Both yeasts and worms hook onto the mucous membrane of the digestive track and suck nutrients from you like vampires.  No matter what you eat and how much you eat, you are malnourished because you are feeding an extended family!  Just think of a country that has limited resources and yet has a large population to feed.**

---

### *Bacterial Infections:*

If yeasts and parasites are Siamese twins, then bacteria is their cousin.  They love to hang out with each other!  After an extensive research, Dr. Livingston-Wheeler (1984) has discovered that all cancer cells contain Progenitor-Cryptocides bacillus.  These bacteria exist in the human body and are usually harmless.  However, when your immunity is weakened, these bacteria can gain a foothold and turn themselves into a lethal cancer microbe in your blood!

When your immune function is low, it's like you have an open-door policy.  All the un-invited guests can come in, whether you like them or not!  Worst of all, these un-invited guests make themselves very comfortable at your home (body) until you decide to get rid of these strangers from within!

*Viral Infections:*

Like bacteria, many viruses stay dormant in the human body and co-exist peacefully. However, when your immune system is weak, every microbial organism in your body will begin to claim its territory. Epstein-Barr virus is a good example. It is said that by age 30, nearly 100% of the population is infected by Epstein-Barr virus (Stoff & Pellegrino, 1992).

People who suffer from diagnoses such as mononucleosis, Crohn's disease, Epstein-Barr virus, candidiasis and Chronic Fatigue Syndrome are usually infected with yeasts, parasites, bacteria and viruses simultaneously. An underweight condition can be a result of feeding all these ever-starving creatures!

## Treatment for Underweight Problems:

Important strategies for correcting the underweight problem include: controlling yeast overgrowth, cleaning up parasites, getting rid of harmful bacteria and viruses, regenerating your digestive function and improving your immunity.

*Herbal Therapy:*

The most important step is to control the harmful overgrowth of yeasts, bacteria and viruses, and to clean up the parasites in your body. Herbal formulas containing goldenseal root, echinacea, dandelion, black walnut hull, burdock, pau d' arco, gotu kola and papaya are often effective in expelling yeasts, parasites, bacteria and viruses.

Some worms can be old and large; therefore, strong formulas and repeated treatment will be needed to weaken their suction hooks and to expel them from the body. Since yeasts and parasites go hand-in-hand, when you find the bodies of parasites in the toilet, you will see a good amount of mucous as well.  This debris usually contains yeasts, bacteria and viruses.

If you are an animal lover, you also need to de-worm your pets. Animals respond well to herbs just like human beings.  Mix cleansing herbal formulas in the pet food.  Make sure that you wash your hands after you pat your pets.  Avoid kissing your pets.  They carry yeasts, parasites, bacteria and viruses all the time.

### *Anti-Yeast Nutritional Approach:*

An anti-yeast nutritional approach with no meats and raw foods is essential to prevent your body from further assaults.  If you crave meats, organically grown chicken from health food stores may be a consideration. Nowadays, many soybean products taste like meat and are rich in protein. Once you change your taste buds, meat cravings will not be a problem any more.

If you must have fish, cold water fish such as salmon, halibut or cod are better choices because they have less chances being infected with yeasts, parasites, bacteria and viruses due to extremely cold water temperatures.

Cook your vegetables.  The heat will kill the yeasts, parasites, bacteria and viruses.  If you must have raw vegetables once in a while, peel the carrot skin and brush the celery under running water very well to make some carrot or celery sticks.  When you learn how to stir-fry your vegetables (see *Healthy and Tasty: Anti-Yeast Cooking*, Tien, 1997), chances are you will not miss your salads (raw vegetables) anymore.  As mentioned previously, slightly cooked vegetables are easier on your digestive system and you can absorb nutrients from them more effectively.

For those of you who want to gain weight, just eat a larger portion of food following the anti-yeast nutritional program.  You may also increase the frequency of food intake.  In between your three meals, snack on healthy, anti-yeast nutritional food if necessary.  The idea is to feed your body with the right food so that your body has a chance to heal and regenerate.

*What is Eating You?*

> **When you are wasting away, you need to pay attention to not only what you are eating physically, but what is eating you emotionally!**

Do a thorough mental check up and follow the instructions in Chapter 11 to release negative emotions which prevent you from having a healthy body and a happy life.

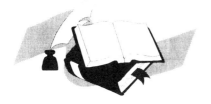

# Chapter 20

# Attention Deficit Disorder (ADD)

*At* least five million Americans have been haunted by symptoms of hyperactivity, short attention-span, distractability, impulsiveness, moodiness, disorganization, learning difficulties, low self-esteem, resistant behavior, irritability, a sense of inadequacy, emotional immaturity and insecurity.

Parents are often frustrated and exhausted by their children with Attention Deficit Disorder (CHADD). Therefore, they tend to rely on medication such as Ritalin, Dexedrine and Cylert for quick relief. Many children suffer from side effects of these stimulants. The side effects range from physical symptoms such as headaches, stomachaches, decreased appetite, skin rash, slow physical growth, high blood pressure or chemical hepatitis to emotional/behavioral symptoms such as depression, social withdrawal, low productivity, insomnia, nightmares or rebound hyperactivity (when the medication wears off).

## Possible Causes of ADD:

In almost three decades of practice, I have found that Attention Deficit Disorder is by far the most complex and elusive disorder among all the emotional/behavioral disorders with which I have dealt. Despite the growing attention this disorder has received in the past few decades, it remains a scientific enigma.

The most widely used diagnostic criteria for ADD can be found in the third revised edition of the Diagnostic and Statistical Manual of Mental Disorders (DSM-III-R). Unfortunately, DSM-III-R has oversimplified ADD by implying that ADD represents a uniform group of patients that are children or adolescents. It states that the onset of behavior usually occurs before the age of seven. My experience reveals that ADD can affect children, adolescents and adults. Each case can differ widely in terms of causes, symptoms, therapeutic process and prognosis.

In an attempt to understand and clarify ADD, scientists have given this disorder many names and causes in the past few decades. Today, the most popularly believed cause for ADD is a biologically and neurologically-based condition which is not due to life experiences or events. This belief has relieved an enormous amount of guilt of many parents and practitioners for not knowing exactly how to deal with patients with ADD. This oversimplified belief has also impeded the therapeutic process from taking place.

After dealing with numerous children and adults with ADD, I have found that the following are common factors. In each case, two or more factors are often present and these factors interact and exacerbate each other.


### *Physical Factors:*

The most common physical factor I have found, which may be shocking to many, is yeast infection involving inner or middle ears. Dr. Harold Levinson in his book, *Total Concentration* (1990) states that more than 80% of the patients with ADD he has seen suffered from inner-ear infections. He explains in great detail how the inner-ear system or the cerebellar-vestibular system (CVS) controls the flow of sensory information entering the brain. When this system is impaired by the infections in the inner ear, our vision, hearing, balance, sense of direction, motion, altitude, depth, smell and anxiety level, and all motor information leaving the brain can be scrambled. Consequently, this auditory drift results in problems in balance and coordination, concentration, memory, hyperactivity and impulsiveness. In some cases, the speech timing is off, which can result in rapid speech or slow, slurred speech. A malfunctioning inner ear has difficulty processing motor input; this in turn makes the affected individual prone to motion-related phobias such as fears of moving elevators, escalators, cars, planes, trains, buses and crowds.

What Dr. Levinson failed to address was what this inner-ear infection is all about and what causes it. In my experience, this inner-ear infection is yeast infection which can be contracted before or after birth.

---

**If a pregnant woman has a yeast infection, she can give this infection to her baby through the blood stream and/or birth canal. The baby can be born with yeast infections manifesting symptoms such as eye or ear infections, respiratory tract congestion and colic.**

---

A person can also contract a yeast infection after birth due to dietary habits, stress and physical environment. This is why there is an adult onset of ADD. In addition to inner-ear yeast infection, another physical factor contributing to ADD is injury, disease or stroke in the frontal lobes of the brain which can result in problems including impulsiveness, poor concentration and disorganization. Injury or disease can happen before, during or after birth. Stroke usually happens during adulthood. According to my experience, this factor accounts for a small percentage of people with ADD.

### *Psychological Factors:*

Most of the children or adults with ADD suffer from psychological distress. The following is a good example:

*Brian, a 12-year-old hispanic male, was brought to my office because of his poor concentration, inability to get along with his siblings and schoolmates, tendency to provoke fights with children and adults, and fluctuating grades. After a few sessions of therapy it became clear that he believed that his birth was a "mistake"; that's why his parents broke up. He firmly believed that he was not loved and not wanted. With counseling, Brian's mother was able to gain insight into his "problem" and learned to interact with Brian in a loving and positive way. In a few weeks, Brian showed marked improvement in his hyperactive and provocative behaviors. His prognosis is good.*

Another example is Kay, a 16-year-old Caucasian high school student.

*Kay was brought to my office because of her impulsive eating, which resulted in overweight problems, poor mental concentration, resistant behavior, constant chattering, rapid speech and low self-esteem. Kay's progress fluctuated during the course of therapy. I attributed this to her parents' attitudes. On the one hand, they wanted Kay to get well. On the other hand, they openly expressed their impatience and readiness to give up on Kay. To complicate the issue further, Kay was adopted. This was not revealed to me until her parents insisted on quitting the therapy because "Kay was not motivated to help herself; therefore, we cannot waste anymore money on her." Kay's prognosis was poor until her parents were willing to participate in the therapy to deal with Kay's complicated emotional issues involving adoption and abandonment.*

## Dietary Factors:

As explained previously, the Standard American Diet (SAD) has created many **sad** stories. Over-consumption of food containing sugar, dairy, wheat, yeast, alcohol, caffeine, nicotine and chemicals (including drugs, food preservatives and coloring, and heavy metal poisoning) has caused every American yeast overgrowth at one time or the other, to a greater or lesser degree. Symptoms of yeast disorder range from head to toe including headaches, poor mental concentration (foggy mind), mid- or inner-ear infections, strep throat, nasal congestion, bloatedness, constipation, diarrhea, skin rash, athlete's foot, mood swings, insomnia, depression and phobias.

*Environmental Factors:*

> **Many people with ADD live in an environment which contributes to or worsens their disorders. Children with ADD often have parents who also suffer from ADD. Some parents recognize their disorders; however, most don't. Many school teachers also have ADD, but most don't recognize or don't want to admit to the affliction.**

In many cases, parents exhibit dysfunctional behavior which worsens their children's ADD. Stress due to parents' divorce, illness, financial hardship, etc., also can complicate a child's ADD.

## Treatment for ADD:

The essence of ADD is that there are no uniform symptoms, causes and treatment modalities. Every case should be given individualized attention and treatment plans. Parents with CHADD need to adjust their expectation of the treatment outcome. Basically, there is no cure for ADD. However, *the symptoms can be controlled* with proper intervention. A combination of psychological counseling, nutritional counseling, Chinese herbal therapy, behavioral modification, biofeedback and sometimes acupuncture and chiropractic can be very effective in symptom control.

*Anti-Yeast Nutritional Therapy:*

An anti-yeast nutritional program works wonders to reduce hyperactivity, poor mental concentration, irritability, moodiness and the other symptoms mentioned above. The logic is very simple: an anti-yeast nutritional program reduces the infection in the middle or inner ear. When the yeast infection is under control, the swelling of tissue goes down. This, in turn, allows sensory input to be transmitted from the external environment to the brain of the recipient without obstacles or blockage. The recipient of this sensory input can then be receptive and responsive.

## *Herbal Therapy:*

Chinese herbal nutrients are also found to be effective in the detoxifying and healing process. The most important formulas to use are the ones that clean up sinus infections.

> **Sinus congestion not only blocks sensory input, but prevents the brain from getting a sufficient supply of oxygen. This, of course, is a double whammy! When the sinus infections are cleared, the mental clarity will also be restored.**

Not every individual with ADD experiences hyperactivity. Some experience low energy and depression. Therefore, additional treatment for uplifting energy and the mood is recommended. Some children also experience digestive problems such as abdominal pain, constipation or diarrhea. Herbal treatment for these symptoms is also necessary to help the individual improve the digestive function.

## *Psychological Counseling:*

As mentioned earlier, all individuals with Attention Deficit Disorder experience emotional issues which have not been worked through. Whether it's children or adults, it is important to identify the core problems contributing to the disorder. Seeking help from experienced therapists dealing with ADD is an essential step.

If impulsiveness is present, the individual will need to be in a behavior modification program either on an individual basis or in a group situation. The purpose of these programs is to help the individual learn to set limits on his or her behavior and learn a new way to gratify needs or delay gratification.

In order to effectively help children with ADD, parents, teachers and therapists need to work together as a team to identify the bottom line issues and to work through them with a conscious effort. One very important step is that parents of children with ADD (or ADHD) and teachers must gain insight into their own "problems" and deliberately work through the issues. In other words, the "helpers" have to seek help before they can really help!

---

**People with ADD are often highly intelligent. They represent too much of a resource for society to waste. Don't give up on them!**

---

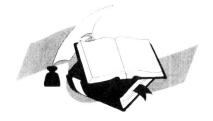

# Chapter 21

# Chronic Fatigue Syndrome (CFS)

———◆———

*Chronic* Fatigue Syndrome (CFS) is an illness characterized by a cluster of symptoms including persistent, recurrent fatigue, headaches, achy muscles, poor digestive function (such as constipation, diarrhea, and bloatedness), low-grade fever, foggy mind, confusion, irritability, lack of motivation and depression.

Both men and women can be affected by Chronic Fatigue Syndrome. In my practice, however, most of the clients are women between the ages of 20 and 50. The personality characteristics of people with Chronic Fatigue Syndrome are highly successful, educated, articulate, and always on the go. Prior to the onset of Chronic Fatigue Syndrome, they were very active with their career activities, and/or were caretakers.

After several years of highly charged activities, they "ran out of gas" and collapsed. These people tended to give, give, give, but did not receive the nurturing which was essential to replenish their reservoir. The "Too Pooped to Pop" (Tien-Hyatt, 1992) feelings are very real to the sufferers. However, most western-trained physicians did not take them seriously.

Some were referred to psychiatrists by their physicians for psychotropic drugs with the reasoning that it was all in their heads!

People with Chronic Fatigue Syndrome have often suffered for many years without a proper diagnosis and treatment. Many of my previous clients had to be on medical disability because they could not carry out regular daily functions which were routine for them before. In some severe cases, daily chores such as brushing teeth or cooking dinner can be taxing for the sufferer.

> **Basically, Chronic Fatigue Syndrome shares similar symptoms with mononucleosis, Epstein-Barr virus, candidiasis, Crohn's disease, and yeast disorders.**

## Causes of Chronic Fatigue Syndrome:

As mentioned earlier, people with Chronic Fatigue Syndrome tend to be high achievers and devoting caretakers. The major causes for their collapse are twofold. The first is what I call "Busy-Taking-Care-of-Others Syndrome." The second is poor dietary habits.

### *Busy-Taking-Care-of-Others Syndrome:*

As mentioned in Chapter 7, many people, especially women, have assumed a caretaking role. They play their roles so well that they often forget about themselves. They are so busy taking care of other people's needs that they don't have time to take care of their own needs. Connie is a good example:

*As a nurse, Connie had been a hard worker in hospitals for more than 10 years. She had been very active in volunteer activities such as the Red Cross or other charity groups. Her mother died of breast cancer when she was five years old. Being the only child, she had been a caretaker for her frail father since she was a teen.*

*Since she was always on the run, she was on the convenient Standard American Diet (SAD) even though she was familiar with what was right for her to eat. The onset of fatigue, headaches, poor mental concentration, weight loss, lack of motivation and depression came slowly in a period of three to six months. Then, she totally collapsed and became bedridden when her boyfriend broke up with her.*

### *Poor Dietary Habits:*

People who are busy taking care of others usually suffer from low self-esteem. When they don't think much of themselves, naturally they don't take good care of themselves. Everybody comes first; they come last. This tendency is also reflected in their dietary habits. Even though Connie was a consulting nutritionist for an outpatient clinic, she did not practice what she preached. Her diet was filled with sugar, dairy, wheat, yeast, alcohol, caffeine and chemicals. Even though she knew she was "allergic" to those kinds of foods, she could not take the time to go to health food stores to shop for the right kinds of foods.

## Treatment for Chronic Fatigue Syndrome:

As explained previously, for any yeast-related health problems, there is no simple treatment. You must be willing to deal with your body and mind at the same time in order to ensure long-lasting results.

## *Energy Boosting:*

The most important step is to boost the energy level so that you can carry on basic activities in your life. An anti-yeast nutritional program is essential to feed your body with the right kind of food and meanwhile, starve the yeasts and parasites which have been partially responsible for this debilitating condition. An anti-yeast nutritional program will control the fermentation and destruction of your cells and tissues. This, in turn, will improve your body's ability to absorb and utilize essential nutrients.

The use of herbal formulas to boost your energy by nourishing the glands and organs such as the thyroid, liver, kidneys and pancreas can be very fruitful. The combination of acupuncture, acupressure, chiropractic, massage or any hands-on-healing technique can be a very helpful supplement to recharge the sluggish "battery."

## *Exercise:*

People with Chronic Fatigue Syndrome can easly sleep 10 to 16 hours a day and still feel fatigued. Exercise will be the last thing they want to do. Remember, yeasts love a still environment that has no air. When your body is immobile, your blood circulation is poor and your oxygen supply is insufficient. This creates an excellent incubator for yeasts to overgrow!

Force yourself to start with five minutes of slow walking around the house or around the block. Slowly increase to 30 minutes a day. You will find that you are invigorated after each slow walk. You will have better results if you walk outdoors. Review the instructions in Chapter 10.

*During the recuperating period, there is one danger to keep in mind. A few days to a few weeks after you get on the right track, you may begin to experience surges of energy. This is an exciting feeling! This excitement often leads you to overdo it again!*

Ellen is a good example:

*After suffering from Chronic Fatigue Syndrome for several years, Ellen was so excited about her "new found energy." Three weeks into the treatment, she woke up one morning with a surge of energy. She quickly resumed the activity level she used to have before the onset of Chronic Fatigue Syndrome. She cleaned the house, did the laundry and grocery shopping, and then went to the gym. While she was working out in the gym, she collapsed and fell on her face!*

---

**Remember the principle of healing? For one year of illness, it takes at least one month to heal. Allow your energy reserve to build up. Don't exhaust your reservor too quickly.**

---

Slow walking is recommended for the first three to six months during the recovery. After that, any vigorous exercise should be introduced slowly, based on your body's ability to handle it.

### *Reestablishing Self-Image:*

*The onset of Chronic Fatigue Syndrome basically is the loss of self.* You need to seek proper professional help to reestablish a sense of self. Many caretakers give their care or love to make themselves feel important and thus feel loved or respected. In order to be loved and respected by others, you must love and respect yourself. See yourself as the most important human being on Earth. *Exercise the art of selfishness. Learn to take care of yourself first before you take care of others.*

Practice self-love and self-respect. Write a brief note or buy a card to praise yourself whenever you accomplish something. Take yourself to a movie or a shopping trip if you feel a little down. Develop a support system with which you can share your joys and agonies. Being a "lone ranger" can be very fatiguing.

Allow yourself to receive love and care. Every so often revert to the child stage to ask for love and attention. If you don't know how, just observe young children. They will show you how you can ask for love and attention without allowing your ego or pride to get in the way.

---

**Chronic Fatigue Syndrome comes from chronic neglect of yourself emotionally and physically. No doctors out there can cure you but yourself. A Chinese proverb says, "A journey of a thousand miles begins with the first step." Take your first step, no matter how hard it is. Each following step will become easier and easier. Sooner or later, you will step out of Chronic Fatigue Syndrome!**

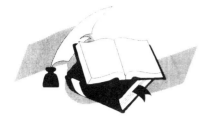

# Chapter 22

# Cancer

———◆———

*Cancer* claims the lives of 272,000 men and 242,000 women every year (Foley & Nechas, 1993). The cost of "treating" (killing and mutilating) cancer patients in the United States alone is over 100 billion dollars a year (Willner,1994). In the past 100 years, cancer research has not made much progress in treating cancer successfully.

## Causes of Cancer:

Many factors have been associated with cancer. Tobacco, alcohol, pollution, an unhealthy work environment, food additives, pesticides, drugs, emotional stress and dietary habits have been cited as the most common factors causing cancer.

*Dietary Factors:*

According to Doll and Peto (1981), the estimated percentage of cancer deaths caused by tobacco was 30%, while that by diet was 35%! Excess dietary fat has been identified as an important contributing factor to colon, liver, gallbladder, breast and endometrial cancers. Ingestion of saccharin and sodium nitrite (food preservatives) have also been associated with cancer. Birth control pills have been reported to contribute to cancers in the female reproductive system.

In nearly three decades of practice, I have found that the same diet which causes yeast disorders also causes cancer! For example, I have noticed that a high incidence of stomach and esophageal cancers among Asian populations is associated with a high intake of fermented, yeast-loaded pickles.

**Dr. Otto Warburg, a Nobel Prize winner in Science in 1931, demonstrates that a cancer cell has the metabolism of a plant cell. He describes the process as "fermentation." A plant cell thrives on carbon dioxide and gives off oxygen as its waste product. This is opposite to the function of "normal cells."**

Other researchers also report that one of the probable mechanisms underlying carcinogenic processes is the cellular release of free oxygen radicals. These free oxygen radicals contribute to DNA damage (Willner, 1994).

Dr. Gaston Naessens, a renowned Canadian biologist in his research for a cancer solution, developed an advanced microscope capable of magnifying 30,000 times (standard microscopes are capable of magnifying 1,800 times). This enabled him to carefully observe an important phenomenon called *polymorphism* (the ability to change form). This is also known as the process of fermentation.

> **When the fermentation process takes place, a cell reverts itself to a more primitive state. This results in more rapid growth and chaos. Moreover, this fermentation process changes the biochemical codes or sensors of the cell.**

The weakened immune system cannot identify the invader and start the normal battle to get rid of this invader. In fact, a weakened immunity may even adopt the identity of the foe (a fermented cancer cell) and attack a normal cell (Willner, 1994).

*Psychological Factors:*

Many researchers assert that we all have cancer genes (oncogenes) in our body. The reason why some get cancer but others don't, is due to the way we handle stressors in our life. *After dealing with numerous cancer clients, I have found that there is symbolic meaning in each type of cancer. For example, women who have breast cancer are usually givers or care-takers. They had been busy giving love and care to others but had not received the nurturing they needed.* In some cases, they craved love and nurturing but did not get it because their husbands had extramarital affairs. Another example is that when a woman has uterine cancer, usually she has unfinished issues regarding sexuality such as sexual molestation or rape. A person who has throat or thyroid cancer usually has unexpressed rage.

**Treatment for Cancer:**

By now, you have a pretty good understanding that poor dietary habits create a chronic situation to incubate cancer cells, and that psychological stress, either chronic or acute, facilitates this incubation process.     The best way to treat or prevent cancer is to deal with the body and mind simultaneously.

### *Anti-Yeast Nutritional Approach:*

The astounding research findings cited previously give you some insight into how the diet causing yeast disorders may also cause cancer!

---

**Hopefully it has become clear to you why it is important to observe the "eight commandments": no sugar, no dairy, no wheat, no yeast, no alcohol, no caffeine, no nicotine and no chemicals.  The first seven items feed yeasts in your body and make the fermentation process more active.  This fermentation process creates abnormal cancer cells. The last item, chemicals, clogs your liver and kidneys and lowers your immunity.**

---

When your immune system is weakened, it can mistake enemies for friends, and vice versa.  A confusing battle can thus begin, either in the form of cancer or autoimmune disease!

### *Psychological Approach:*

Cancer is a life-threatening illness and an extremely traumatic experience.  You can allow the illness to consume you or you can take the bull by the horns and fight back!  *Many people exercise their informed freedom of choice and are able to create a "permanent remission." If you don't see cancer as a sentence, but a new beginning, chances are you can win the battle and claim victory.*

Dr. Bernie Siegel, in his book, *Peace, Love & Healing* (1989), advocates "self-induced healing." He believes that feelings are natural chemicals that can heal or kill. As a medical doctor, he chooses to help his cancer patients use these natural chemicals to cure and heal themselves. "Anything that offers hope has the potential to heal including thoughts, suggestions, symbols and placebos." As a result of this firm belief, he has helped countless cancer patients create miracle cures!

The late Norman Cousins, in his book, *Anatomy of an Illness* (1985), suggested that if you have a highly developed purpose, a strong will to live and a creative way of living, you will have a potent healing force! By exercising this healing force, together with laughter, courage and tenacity, he successfully fought against a crippling disease and increased his longevity.

Crisis in Chinese is 危機. 危 means danger. 機 means opportunity. When there is danger, there is also an opportunity! Once you decide to take advantage of the opportunity to start a new life which is more functional for you, your bodily functions may change quickly. After you have made a conscious decision to live a better life, there are several things you can do to facilitate this process. They include: meditation, affirmation, prayers, releasing negative energy and finishing unfinished business.

### *Meditation:*

Regular meditation at least once a day for 10 to 30 minutes is a wonderful way to manage your stress, improve your mental clarity and concentration, and improve your blood circulation. Most people inflicted with cancer "think too much!" Follow the meditation technique detailed in Chapter 11 to unwind and empty your mind on a regular basis. The meditation process can generate endorphins, a natural chemical in your body to reduce pain and to give you a high, yet calm feeling. This feeling can help you combat cancer!

I have been meditating regularly for more than 20 years. Many times I have gotten miraculous answers to my questions during meditation. Meditation allows you to be in touch with your higher self. Your higher self (or your subconscious mind) has the innate intelligence to heal yourself on physical, emotional and spiritual levels.

---

**Cancer is simply a warning that you need healing on all levels. Through meditation, it may become clear to you what path you should take in the healing process!**

---

*Affirmation:*

I often share the following affirmation with my clients or anyone I know:

*"I am whole, perfect, strong, powerful, harmonious, loving, giving, loved, wealthy, healthy and happy!"*

This affirmation can be very powerful if you repeat it 300 times a day! That's right. Three hundred times a day! Squeaky wheels get greased first. If you say this affirmation from the bottom of your heart at least 300 times a day, you will obligate the universe to offer what you ask for! In my book, *Being the Best You Can Be -- A Practical Guide for Harmony and Prosperity* (1996), I cited a previous client of mine who used this technique diligently and received $5,000 in a most miraculous way. When you are faced with a life-threatening disease such as cancer, be generous in your affirmations. Remember, it's free of charge! What are you waiting for?!

***Prayers:***

If you believe in God, any kind of God, pray! Even if you don't believe in God, I still urge you to pray. Again, it's free of charge. What have you got to lose?! I have been praying on my knees at least twice a day, once in the morning when I roll out of bed and again in the evening before I go to bed. Praying on your knees makes you humble. Cancer is a very humbling experience. When you can reduce yourself to a humbling capacity, that's the time you will get the most miraculous effect!

I often suggest my cancer clients say the following prayers.

Prayer in the morning:

*"Dear God,*

*Thank you for bringing me another wonderful day! Today please make it a very healing and productive day. Please bring me the best resources I need to heal myself on physical, emotional and spiritual levels. Please fill my heart with love, joy and positive attention. Thank you, thank you, thank you!"*

Prayer in the evening:

*"Dear God,*

*Thank you for helping me to live through another wonderful day. Today I have... (recount your accomplishments). Please continue to give me strength and guidance to achieve perfect health and happiness. Thank you, thank you, thank you!"*

No matter how you feel, always start with positive notes in the morning and end with positive notes in the evening. Only focus on positive thinking. Never waste any energy on negative thinking!

> **The internal reality you create for yourself through prayers can override the external reality. If it is difficult for you to pray to God, pray to the universe or your higher self. Remember one cardinal principle: practice makes perfect!**

### *Releasing Negative Energy:*

Without exceptions, all cancer clients I have encountered carry anger, resentment, grief, regret and guilt to a greater or lesser degree. As explained previously, carrying these negative emotions is just like driving your car with the hand brake on. Not only do you have to press the gas pedal harder to move the car, but you cause a lot of wear and tear to the car. It is obvious that these negative emotions drag down your immunity! It is of ultimate importance, therefore, to release these negative emotions as soon as possible!

Follow the technique in Chapter 13. You can do this while you are meditating in a quiet place, or while you are driving. Make sure you keep your eyes open if you are doing this while you are driving. Here are some important steps:

1. Go through the deep breathing procedure and release tension from toe to head.
2. Mentally connect your first chakra to the center of the earth with an imaginary golden rope.
3. Turn on the switch in your seventh chakra and light up the center of your head. Claim your territory in this sacred space.
4. Surround your entire body with an 18-inch-thick ring of oval-shaped golden light.
5. Put a rose outside of the golden light and in front of you. Put in it your worry or concern about your cancer condition or other issues such as finances, family, relationships, etc. Blow up that concern with the rose,

one concern at a time. Everything turns into golden dust. As these golden particles come down on you, they reinforce the existing 18-inch thick golden light and give you more positive energy! Repeat this procedure as many times as you want until you feel relieved or more comfortable.

The whole procedure only takes one to two minutes to finish once you become experienced with it. Every day when you drive to and from work or stay at home, instead of worrying about your illnesses, use your time constructively by releasing negative energy and bringing about the positive outcome you wish!

## *Finish Unfinished Business:*

Whether you believe in reincarnation or not, or whether you are going to die or live, it is important that you finish your unfinished business. Remember we are all living and dying at the same time. Nobody has a crystal ball to predict when your number is up. Pretend that you only have six months to live; what would like to take care of quickly so that when you check out, you are nice and clean?

If you are a procrastinator or you are always behind schedule, this is a good chance for you to catch up! Make a list of things that you really want to accomplish in this lifetime and start working on the priority items. Among your priority items should be the releasing of your anger, resentment, grief, regret and guilt toward any person who is alive or deceased. Use the format in Chapter 7 to write a releasing letter to the persons you want to address. If you feel too weak or confused to do this alone, seek professional help from a competent health practitioner.

> *I cannot guarantee that the information contained in this book can save your life. However, I can guarantee that if you follow every suggestion I make in this book diligently, you will live or die more comfortably!*

Hilda is an example.

*When Hilda was brought to my office by a friend who had been listening to my radio shows in southern California, she was terminally ill with liver cancer. She was well aware that cancer had metastasized to her stomach, lungs and spine. Her neck was also covered by various-sized tumors which were burned and charcoaled by radiation. She had difficulty breathing and keeping food down. On our first session, I explained to her my philosophy and treatment strategies. She liked them and agreed to cleanse her system as much as possible during her final days.*

*I first put her on an anti-yeast nutritional program containing mostly brown rice gruel with beans, peas, and carrots, something easy for a weak digestive system to digest and absorb. I also put her on heavy duty cleansing herbs in tea and capsule form. Two weeks later she came back for a follow- up session. She told me a "gross" story. She had passed an approximately five-foot long feces with tarry black color. The swelling of her stomach went down and the tumors on her neck miraculously disappeared! Her skin color looked much better than it had during the first visit. Obviously, she was full of toxins from severe constipation, radiation and chemotherapy!*

*She had more energy at this time and was willing to go through a heavy-duty emotional cleansing process. I explained to her that liver cancer is an indication of unresolved anger and resentment. She quickly revealed that 35 years ago, her husband left her with two small children for another woman who was supposed to have had more wild and exciting sex with him. She took this as a tremendous insult since she was regarded as a beautiful and sexy woman by many. Carrying much anger and resentment, she struggled to raise her children alone. When her two beautiful daughters were grown, her husband returned.*

*Even though she maintained peace with her husband on the surface, inside she was still trembling with rage. Along with years of financial struggle and poor nutrition, her body finally broke down. She was guided to write a letter to her husband to release her hidden anger and resentment. Even though she did not give the letter to her husband, the process of writing the letter gave her a chance for catharsis. As a result, she became stronger and learned how to talk back whenever her husband behaved like a bully. She died three months later. Before she died, the pain in her stomach had been greatly reduced by the herbal formulas that she used both internally and externally. She was also able to gain a sense of control and peace during her passing.*

Anita's case has a happy ending:

*While attending a party in Houston, Anita passed out. After being rushed to the hospital for a thorough examination, it was found that she had a tumor in her brain about the size of a golf ball. Her sister had been listening to my radio shows in southern California and urged her to consult with me. I suggested that she go ahead with surgery as had been scheduled. However, after the surgery, she should come to Los Angeles for healing and recovery.*

*Shortly after surgery, she took the train from Houston to Los Angeles to start a new life. I quickly put her on the anti-yeast nutritional program and started her on a heavy dosage of herbal therapy. The first three months she was taking 107 tablets and capsules of herbal formulas per day, upon my insistence. The dosage was tapered off thereafter. Luckily her surgeon in Houston was not against herbal medicine. He actually left Anita in my hands completely. In addition to using the anti-yeast nutritional approach and herbal therapy, I also worked heavily with Anita on her emotional issues. Basically, her husband was the major cause of her brain tumor! Being a flight attendant, Anita had a habit of pleasing everybody, including her husband. Every time she disagreed with her husband on an issue, he would pull out a gun and point it at her head. This had gone on for many years and she just kept the fear and secret to herself. Finally, her body could not take it anymore and gave her a life-threatening warning!*

*During the course of psychological counseling, I invited Anita's husband to join us for a few sessions. He finally agreed to grant her a divorce. After six months of intensive therapy (once or twice per week), Anita had become a more assertive person, got the divorce settled, grew back her hair (her hair was shaved off for the brain surgery), found a new, loving boyfriend (who later became her husband), and got a clean bill of health!*

*Although Anita's family was able to give her a lot of emotional support during her recovery, they were not able to give her any financial support. When Anita ran out of funds, she began to sell her jewelry, watches and cars to continue to support herself and the treatment. Her determination to fight this battle greatly impressed me. When she was totally out of funds, I hired her as a part-time secretary to work off the balance she owed for the therapy.*

At the time of this writing, it has been nine years since I last saw Anita. I have spoken with her on the phone from time to time in the past nine years, and she still has a clean bill of health!

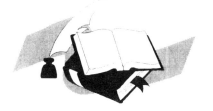

# Chapter 23

# Acquired Immune Deficiency Syndrome (AIDS)

———◆———

*Acquired* Immune Deficiency Syndrome (AIDS) has generated many controversial issues in the past 1-1/2 decades. Let's carefully examine each issue.

## What Is AIDS?

Acquired Immune Deficiency Syndrome (AIDS) is a cluster of symptoms indicating that there is an immune deficiency in the body. Therefore, AIDS is not a disease; it is a collection of immune deficiency symptoms signaling that your body's defense is weak.

## Does HIV Cause AIDS?

Since Dr. Robert Gallo, a retrovirologist with the National Cancer Institute claimed in 1980 that the human retrovirus (HTLM-1) is the cause of AIDS, the whole nation has been stormed by fear and confusion. Dr. Willner in his book, **Deadly Deception** (1994), provided heavily documented proof that HIV does not cause AIDS. The human retrovirus is a kind of virus that is dormant or inactive. Its replication and survival is totally dependent on the viability of the host cell. If the host cell dies, the virus is finished. However, Dr. Gallo and his cohorts have painted the picture that this type of virus can attack or infiltrate the human immune system at such a high speed that the destruction process could never be detected by modern technology. Therefore, this cannot-be-found virus is "mysterious" and all-powerful, and has claimed 100,000 lives in the past 10 years in a scary AIDS "epidemic."

On April 23, 1984, Dr. Gallo announced that he had discovered a new kind of virus called HTLV-III, inferring that it was a member of the family of retroviruses he had previously discovered. His claim was bolstered by Margaret Heckler, Secretary of the Department of Health and Human Services, who was under great pressure to come up with some answer to the looming "epidemic." "Today we add another miracle to the long honor roll of American medicine and science," said Heckler. Together with Dr. Gallo, they promised that we would have a vaccine within two years. That very day, Dr. Gallo filed a U.S. patent for an HIV test kit which has made him very wealthy. Margaret Heckler also very quickly awarded the lucrative contract for AZT to Burroughs-Wellcome Pharmaceutical Company before the first scientific paper on it ever appeared in any U.S. journal.

In 1987, Dr. Peter Duesberg, an internationally renowned retrovirologist with the University of California at Berkeley, published an article in **Cancer Research** which badly shook the foundation of the HIV-AIDS theory. Risking his job, reputation and grants, this Nobel Prize nominee maintained his position and committed to the truth. Recently, more than 500 of the world's most prominent scientists banded together and formed the "Group for the Scientific Reappraisal of the HIV-AIDS Hypothesis." The founder of this group is Dr. Charles A. Thomas, a Harvard molecular biologist.

## How Does AIDS Get Transmitted?

The propoganda has been that people with AIDS carry a deadly virus called HIV. This scary, almighty HIV is transmitted through bodily fluids such as saliva and semen. Therefore, kissing and sexual intercourse are dangerous activities because they can transmit HIV. Since HIV is a dormant, harmless virus in the human body, it is not contagious.

When a person has AIDS, his or her immune system is so low that all the opportunistic organisms such as harmful yeasts, bacteria, viruses and parasites can claim their territories in the body.

> **Consequently, after you have sex with a person who has AIDS, you may experience an instant flare-up comprising of trench mouth, sore throats, fatigue and vaginal or rectal itch. Yes! Yeast infections can be transmitted sexually and you may experience yeast disorder symptoms within 24 hours after the sexual encounter!**

If your body is already incubating a severe case of yeast disorders, even if you just feed your body with yeast favorite foods such as sugar, dairy, wheat, yeast, alcohol, caffeine, nicotine and chemicals (drugs), you will experience the same kind of symptoms without any sexual encounter! Of course, with a sexual partner who has AIDS, it will certainly become a double whammy! *Many people have mistaken the transmission of yeast infections for that of HIV infections.*

## How Did Magic Johnson Get Infected with AIDS and Will He Die of AIDS?

Magic Johnson (the basketball superstar) was said to have had at least 400 sexual partners up to this point. He also had a very hectic lifestyle. He did not have a proper diet and proper amount of rest. Although he might not openly admit it, chances are he was on recreational drugs. All these were risk factors for AIDS.

Will he die of AIDS? Nobody has a crystal ball. The answer lies within him. If he were to make a drastic change in his lifestyle, he certainly would have a chance to survive and thrive. These positive changes include: an anti-yeast nutritional program, herbal therapy, monogamy, a proper amount of sleep and rest, and cessation of all drugs and alcohol, including AZT!

By the way, if his wife has a case of yeast disorder, she would also need to be treated. This would reduce his chances of getting more yeasts from sexual activities with his wife. This advice applies to all people with AIDS and their monogamous sexual partners!

## How Did Arthur Ashe Get Infected with AIDS?

Arthur Ashe (the famous tennis star) received blood transfusions through surgery. Remember, yeast disorders can be transmitted through the blood stream, birth canal, sexual contact and any exposure to yeasts. Up to date there is no procedure sophisticated enough to detect yeast disorders in the blood. Arthur Ashe might have gotten AIDS from blood which was loaded with yeasts, but not "infectious HIV!"

On top of that, if he was under heavy emotional stress and having a hectic lifestyle, his immune system did not have a good chance to restore its function. Again, the solution is simple: do everything to rebuild the immune system but do not take AZT!

## How Do Babies Get Infected with AIDS?

We certainly cannot blame babies for promiscuity or homosexuality. All AIDS-infected babies that have been brought to my office (starting at two-weeks-old) have one thing in common: their mothers were heavy drug-users! Most of them were cocaine or heroine babies. Just picture the starving babies in Africa. This is how these babies with AIDS looked like! These babies suffered from a severe case of malnutrition and yeast disorders! Their symptoms included fever, colic, poor feeding and sleep patterns, seizures and growth retardation. And please don't feed these babies with AZT!

## What is AZT?

AZT (azidothymidine) had been sitting on the shelf since the 1960s during Nixon's "war on cancer." It was an experimental drug that failed as a cancer remedy because it was too toxic to use. AZT was a drug in search of a disease, and it found AIDS at an opportune time!

---

**AZT is a random killer of infected and healthy cells. Like antibiotics, it kills both bad guys and good guys. It even kills T-cells and B-cells (our immune cells) and red blood cells (that carry oxygen). AZT is a chain terminator of the DNA synthesis of all cells. In the long run, it kills the person! Unfortunately, some 180,000 people are now being treated with AZT!**

---

What are the side effects of AZT besides killing your cells? They include: cancer, hepatitis, poor mental concentration, hyperactivity, seizures, anxiety, depression, irritability, generalized aches and pains, anemia, leukopenia, impotence, nausea, chest pain, difficulty breathing, insomnia, vertigo, and muscle atrophy (wasting away). If you compare this list with the yeast disorder symptoms in Chapter 5, you will find that the majority of them coincide! *So far as I know, all the AIDS clients who were on heavy dosages and prolonged use of AZT died. Their symptoms of immune deficiency were worsened by AZT and their deaths were hastened by severe yeast disorders facilitated by AZT!*

## Do We Have an AIDS Epidemic?

The press has undoubtedly contributed to this "epidemic." In comparison, the number of people who died of AIDS is far smaller than that of automobile accidents, iatrogenic diseases, cancer and cardiovascular diseases. Each year, automobile accidents kill more than 60,000 people; iatrogenic diseases (disease caused by doctors) kills 12,000; cancer kills over 450,000; and heart disease kills over 750,000. However, AIDS kills approximately 10,000 each year. Which one is the "epidemic?"

The World Health Organization (WHO) has reported that the conversion rate from HIV-positive to AIDS for the United States is 1.5%; Zaire, .004% (350 cases of AIDS out of three million of HIV-positive), and Haiti, 0.1% (912 cases of AIDS out of 360,000 HIV-positive). Africa and Haiti have been blamed as the source of "import" for HIV. At the rate mentioned above, it will take 75 to 100 years to kill the current batch of individuals who are HIV-positive in the U.S.; 25,000 years in Zaire; and 1,000 years in Haiti! It is actually safer for you to move to Zaire or Haiti if you are worried about the AIDS "epidemic!"

## Causes of AIDS:

What really caused AIDS then? In the past 1-1/2 decades, I have found the following characteristics are common among the AIDS, ARC (AIDS-related-complex) or HIV-positive clients with whom I have dealt:

1. Poor dietary habits (malnutrition)
2. Using recreational drugs heavily
3. Promiscuity
4. Poor self-image
5. Emotional conflicts with family due to homosexuality
6. Unstable relationships with lover(s)

In most cases, all six characteristics are present. In some, at least four or more.

## *Poor Dietary Habits:*

Without exception, all the AIDS, ARC and HIV-positive clients who came to my office suffered from malnutrition. The majority of them were gay men who didn't cook. They ate out most of the time. The Standard American Diet (SAD), of course, created many sad stories. Many of them also partied a lot. The common party foods were pizza, beer, chips, etc. Some also didn't eat regular meals. They ate only when they had time or felt like it.

## *Using Recreational Drugs Heavily:*

Again, without exception, they all had used recreational drugs heavily at one time or the other. The most common is marijuana (I was not surprised when Proposition 215 was passed in California in November 1996! Almost every American client I know used marijuana at one time or the other, to a greater or lesser degree). Many of them also use "poppers" (amyl nitrite). They shared the inhaler at parties to boost their sexual energy and to intensify orgasms, especially in a group sex situation. Some of them are also on multiple drugs such as LSD, heroine and cocaine. Use of alcohol (mostly beer), of course, is part of the routine!

## *Promiscuity:*

Many have just come out of the closet and feel a sense of liberation. According to my clients, it is not unusual for a gay man to go to three or four parties a night and be engaged in sexual activities with multiple sexual partners in one night. The use of condoms, of course, is inconvenient. Even though they do not catch HIV through sexual activities, they can catch yeast infections and other sexually transmitted diseases through kissing and intercourse.

## *Poor Self-Image:*

To a greater or lesser degree, every homosexual client I had encountered suffered a poor self-image. The following is an example:

> *John, a corporate executive, had to wear a ring to pretend that he was a married man. When invited to a party with his "wife," he would always decline the offer by saying that his "wife" did not like parties. He always dashed out of his office at five o'clock for fear that his colleagues might invite him to social functions and find out that he was gay.*

A sense of inadequacy and being an outcast is often prevalent with both gay men and women. This long-term emotional burden naturally affects their immunity in a negative way!

## *Emotional Conflicts with Family Due to Homosexuality:*

Most of them realized their homosexual tendency since childhood. However, they tried hard to hide their homosexuality all their lives, until they got AIDS. Before the onset of AIDS, some even forced themselves to get married and have children. However, the real joy they had was with their homosexual lovers instead of their wives or children. This, of course, caused broken marriages and a lot of conflicts. Even for those who remained single, it was difficult to discuss their sexual preference with their family. A chronic state of emotional stress thus ensued.

### *Unstable Relationships with Lovers:*

Many homosexual men have multiple sexual partners. When the AIDS scare broke out, they began to stabilize their relationship with one partner to limit their chances of getting AIDS. However, emotionally speaking, they were not happy. My observation of the homosexual clients I have encountered seems to show that they were more apt to change partners than their heterosexual counterparts. Relationships can be rewarding, yet they also can be draining. A frequent change of partners requires a lot of energy and time, and leads to feelings of instability.

## Treatment for AIDS:

For 20 years, American researchers have spent hundreds of billions of dollars looking for one single virus responsible for a complex illness such as cancer. They have found nothing! History is repeating itself. We are now making the same mistake in AIDS research and treatment.

The mentality of Americans has been looking for "a quick fix." Take two tablets of aspirin or Tylenol and the headache will be gone in 30 minutes.

---

**Instead of taking the responsibility to eradicate dysfunctional habits and develop functional ones, Americans like to find some kind of virus to place the blame on, and then use the vaccine created from that virus to cure the disease. The reason why the AIDS conspiracy has gone so far is because Dr. Gallo and his cohorts simply took advantage of this mentality.**

---

*Remember the Toyota advertisement?  "You've asked for it; you got it!"*

Treating AIDS is like treating cancer; it requires a total lifestyle change!  For those who have survived and thrived, they did just that!  Those who relied on a quick fix such as AZT died more quickly and miserably than they would have liked.  The following are treatment methods I have found helpful to those who have made a conscious decision to live.

### *Anti-Yeast Nutritional Approach:*

It goes without saying that an anti-yeast nutritional approach should be employed.  *Over the years I have found that when people have AIDS, cancer, lupus, or a severe case of yeast disorder, they emit the same type of body odor.  Their bodies have fermented!  The best way to reduce or stop this fermentation process is to not feed the yeasts in your body with their favorite foods.*

For babies with AIDS, just prepare food as for adults and then grind the food with some boiled purified water in a food processor.

### *Stopping Drugs, Alcohol and Cigarettes Immediately:*

Drug, alcohol and nicotine addictions have been known to be difficult to cease.  Fortunately, when people are confronted with the life-or-death issue, they are more willing to quit cold turkey on these addictions.  Drugs alter and decrease the immune function of your cells.  They also clog your liver and kidneys and further lower your immunity.  Recreational drugs have been responsible for destroying the immune system rapidly.  Topped with the extremely toxic effects of AZT, you will not have a chance to survive.  Therefore, stop taking AZT!  Review Chapter 10 again to refresh your memory regarding the "eight commandments."

### *Herbal Therapy:*

Sometimes your body is so starved, an anti-yeast nutritional program alone is not enough to restore your strength. As with my cancer clients, I usually put all of my AIDS clients on heavy-duty herbal treatment. The concentrated herbal nutrients are essential to "recharge the battery" when it's nearly dead! This, of course, creates a heavy-duty cleansing process. Especially for those who have Kaposi's sarcoma, the skin condition can get worse before it gets better. Headaches are also common during the cleansing crisis because of withdrawal from drugs, alcohol or nicotine. With AIDS, the cleansing crisis usually comes and goes like waves. Sometimes a "tidal wave" may come and you may feel like you were being run over by a truck. This is a good sign. This means the herbal therapy is working effectively!

For babies with AIDS, open a capsule and pour the herbal content into the baby's formula or mix with baby food. Most babies actually appear to enjoy the "herbal cocktail!"

### *Coming to Terms with Homosexuality:*

Counseling is essential to help people with AIDS, ARC and HIV-positive to come to terms with their homosexuality. Through counseling countless homosexual clients both in Taiwan and the United States, I have found that homosexual individuals were born with the homosexual tendency. Most homosexuals realized that they were gay when they were young children. Because of stigma, they tried to hide their homosexuality and "behave" like heterosexual individuals. Of course, it takes a lot of energy to deal with such a secret conflict.

> **The pressure to be "normal" comes from the expectations of family and society. Society as a whole needs to realize that when people are born with homosexuality, it is just like people who are born with diabetes. They are different and require a different lifestyle. However, being different is not equal to being inferior. Respect the difference and let them be!**

Homosexual individuals also need to project a more confident image. Once you feel strong inside, you will not allow anyone to point the stick at you and place a negative label on you. Discrimination is everywhere. However, you don't have to be a victim! There have been people that try hard to correct my accent so that I can speak like a typical American. I have decided to keep my accent so that I can sound like a typical Chinese-American. I am proud of being a Chinese-American and proud of being different! As long as you can make a valuable contribution to your family and society, who cares if you came from a homosexual community or from a different planet?!

### *Activating a Support System:*

Many homosexual individuals are loners mostly because of years of alienation from their families. When full-blown AIDS occurs, some will return to their families for care, while others will die in the presence of their lovers without their family members. A Chinese custom asserts that the best way to die is in the middle of your living room, while surrounded by all of your family members (              ). This implies that support is important whether you live or die. This support system should be developed whether you have AIDS or not!

Many people turn to AIDS support groups. The downside of this support group is that most of the group members see themselves as victims. They often look for a rescuer but don't realize that the rescuer lies within themselves. Fear of death is so strong that the atmosphere of the group is often depressing, especially when group leaders announce the death toll of each week or month. Another problem is that group members share information with each other in terms of which physician in town has grants and can offer a free supply of AZT. What is heartbreaking to me is that many have responded very well to holistic treatment, then all of a sudden they drop the natural, holistic treatment and rush to a physician for AZT.

*I ask, "Why?"*
*The reply: "Because, it is free!"*
*I ask, "Do you want to die for free?"*
*Silence.*

**Many did die for free!  It took me awhile to accept that it was their karma.  There was nothing I could do when they chose not to take the responsibility to live!**

Those who survived AIDS are the ones who activated their entire family support system and got holistic treatment without using AZT or other drugs such as interferon (another experimental drug used by some physicians for AIDS). When family members are involved, in addition to emotional support, they may offer financial support for treatment or rides to and from the doctor's office. They are also inclined to fix meals following an anti-yeast nutritional program as suggested. Every bit of support helps when the individual is extremely weak  physically and emotionally!

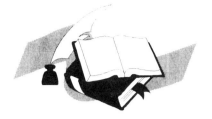

# Chapter 24

# Diabetes

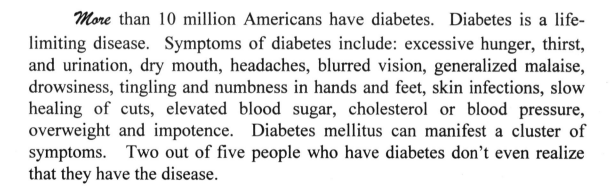

*More* than 10 million Americans have diabetes. Diabetes is a life-limiting disease. Symptoms of diabetes include: excessive hunger, thirst, and urination, dry mouth, headaches, blurred vision, generalized malaise, drowsiness, tingling and numbness in hands and feet, skin infections, slow healing of cuts, elevated blood sugar, cholesterol or blood pressure, overweight and impotence. Diabetes mellitus can manifest a cluster of symptoms. Two out of five people who have diabetes don't even realize that they have the disease.

## Types of Diabetes:

There are two types of diabetes. The cause of Type I (or juvenile) diabetes is the inability of the pancreas to produce ample insulin. Insulin is a hormone formed in the Islets of Langerhans in the pancreas. The function of insulin is to carry blood sugar into cells. Thus, our cells have an energy source. Type I (juvenile) diabetes is usually developed during childhood. This is a serious type of diabetes, and children are often discouraged from exercising to avoid overexertion. As a result, they tend to develop heart, eye and kidney problems later in life. Because they are dependent on regular injections of insulin, they also experience severely damaged blood vessels.

Another type is adult-onset Type II diabetes. This type usually produces sufficient insulin. However, this insulin does not function properly in transporting glucose (blood sugar) and nutrients into cells. This type of diabetes is usually controllable by diet, exercise and stress management.

Both types of diabetes are associated with degenerative diseases such as cardiovascular problems, digestive disorders and liver dysfunction. The bottom line cause is malnutrition!

## Treatment for Diabetes:

> **Treatment for both Type I (juvenile) and Type II (adult-onset) are basically the same. The bottom line is to nourish the body, so that the quantity and quality of insulin production will be improved!**

The combination of an anti-yeast nutritional program, herbal therapy, exercise and stress management usually works wonders for diabetes.

### *Anti-Yeast Nutritional Program:*

As discussed in Chapters 6 and 10, sugar is a favorite food of yeasts. Yeasts thrive instantly in the presence of sugar! The unused blood sugar in the body will certainly give yeasts a big feast! On top of that, if you put more yeast-favorite foods into your body, can you imagine what a wonderful party they are going to have!  An anti-yeast nutritional program is thus essential to control the tremendous overgrowth of yeasts in your body when you have diabetes!  An anti-yeast nutritional program can also lower blood sugar, blood pressure and cholesterol substantially within  just a few weeks.

Carmen is a good example:

*As a business woman,  Carmen travelled a lot. When she was on the road, it was very difficult for her to eat meals regularly.  She ate when she had time.  The content of the foods she ate, of course, consisted of the Standard American Diet (SAD).  In addition to having adult-onset diabetes, she was also overweight and hypertensive.*

*Whenever she was in town for a few weeks, she would come to my office for our ready-made frozen food, anti-yeast vegetarian cuisine.  Even though I encourage people to cook fresh foods, for those who hardly have time to eat, let alone cook, this frozen food is considered the second best.  Every time she had our frozen food, her blood sugar would drop from over 300 to around 150 and her blood pressure would stabilize.  She also reduced her weight at an average of two pounds per week.*

### Herbal Therapy:

The strategy is to use concentrated herbal nutrients to nourish the entire system, especially the pancreas, adrenal glands, liver, and thyroid.  When your entire system functions well, the pancreas, adrenal glands, liver and thyroid work together harmoniously to release various hormones to maintain a steady blood sugar level.

The pancreas has multiple functions.  1) It produces and secretes enzymes to metabolize foods and to convert complex carbohydrates to simple sugars. 2) It releases a bicarbonate fluid to maintain a proper acid/alkaline balance in the digestive tract. 3) It produces insulin to transport sugar into cells. 4) It produces a hormone called glucagon which raises your blood sugar level, and thus supresses your appetite. Your adrenal gland releases adrenaline, which stimulates the release of glycogen (sugar stored in the liver and muscles). Your thyroid releases the hormone thyroxine, which metabolizes all foods.

---

**As you can see, the process of sugar metabolism is very complicated and delicate. If any part of the function is impaired, the chain operation can become inefficient. It is important, therefore, to nourish the organs and glands simultaneously to ensure efficient and effective sugar metabolism.**

---

Herbal formulas geared toward the restoration of the function of the pancreas, adrenal glands, liver, thyroid, and the entire digestive system are therefore essential. In severe cases, acupuncture should be considered to "recharge the battery."

*Exercise:*

It is common sense that exercise burns the excess sugar in the body, and thus reduces the amount of insulin required to lower the blood sugar level. Excess blood sugar can result in ketosis and coma. It is a life-threatening condition! Regular exercise also facilitates blood circulation. This, in turn, can prevent gangrene in the lower extremities. Gangrene is a condition in which tissue starves to death because of a poor supply of blood and nutrients. On top of that, the opportunistic yeasts will take advantage of the situation and cause stubborn infections of the skin. This is not uncommon among severe cases of diabetes.

As mentioned previously, slow walking is an excellent type of excercise for all ages, and free of charge! You do not have to go to the gym even if you don't have the money or time. Thirty minutes of slow walking around the block every day will improve your circulation, digestive function, energy and mental clarity. *The more tired you feel, the more necessary it is for you to start with gentle exercise, such as slow walking.*

*Stress Management:*

By now, you are aware that stress plays an important role in every aspect of your health. Since diabetes is a condition which requires constant "watch," a regular stress management technique such as meditation or self-hypnosis is very helpful. Especially those of you who have hypertension in addition to diabetes, stress management can do wonders to lower your blood pressure.

---

**Diabetes involves the deterioration of multiple glands and organs; therefore, you do need an "overhaul"! Don't wait until you need amputation or are completely impotent to start taking care of yourself. Drop your denial mechanism and start a new lifestyle now!**

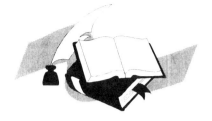

# Chapter 25

# Premenstrual Syndrome (PMS)

———◆———

*Premenstrual* Syndrome is a cluster of symptoms experienced by women about seven to ten days before their periods. These symptoms include: headaches, poor mental concentration, mood swings, depression, anxiety, irritability, crying spells, bloatedness, breast tenderness, fatigue, sugar cravings, water retention, muscle aches in the lower extremities, pelvic discomfort or pain, insomnia, skin breakout, weight gain and loss of sexual desire.

From puberty to menopause, every woman experiences premenstrual syndrome at one time or another, to a lesser or greater degree. About 40% of women experience noticeable and consistent symptoms. Some are so severe that every month they are paralyzed by pain and emotional disturbance. Kathy is an example:

*At least one week before every period, Kathy felt like a basket case. Her mental confusion, depression, anxiety and irritability was so severe that she had to call in sick to work and stay home. She was phobic about seeing anyone. Staying home was also easier when she needed to binge on sugary foods. Her entire body bloated like a balloon. Cramps often made her bed-ridden. She was very angry with this debilitating disease, but the only thing she could do was crying about it. After her period came, she would find that she gained at least five pounds in each cycle!*

***Premenstrual syndrome can also affect relationships. One time a husband brought in his wife to me and said, "You fix my wife. Otherwise, either she will kill me, or I will kill her!" The wife nodded her head and agreed.***

## Causes of PMS:

About seven to ten days before each period, there are biochemical changes in a woman's body. Hormones such as prostaglandin, estrogen, progesterone and prolactin escalate. These hormones increase the blood volume. Consequently, symptoms of water retention, bloatedness, weight gain and sugar cravings follow.

> **Why sugar cravings? When blood volume increases, the amount of blood sugar also increases. Remember, your little friends, yeasts, are always waiting for an opportunity to have a party. The increased amount of blood sugar is just what they need!**

After they are well fed with sugar, they want more! They cry out, "Feed me! Feed me!" If you don't understand what is going on, and feed them with more sugar, then you become the victim of a losing battle! Yeast overgrowth symptoms will thus take a toll on you.

What is the cause of all these hormonal changes? Why is it that some women are debilitated every month, but others don't even know they've got their periods until their panties are stained? It is the same old story: malnutrition and long term physical and emotional stress.

## Treatment for PMS:

Luckily, for every problem there is a natural solution! By now, you probably have already figured out my formulas for treating PMS.

### *Anti-Yeast Nutritional Approach:*

As you can see, yeast disorders can exacerbate a lot of physical and emotional illnesses. In the case of PMS, because of the particular tendency toward sugar cravings, it is of ultimate importance to stay on an anti-yeast nutritional program if you want to gain control. Don't wait until the premenstrual period to get on the anti-yeast nutritional program. The anti-yeast nutritional program should be followed all year along to prevent the occurrence of PMS.

---

**Feed your body with complex carbohydrates instead of simple sugars. Complex carbohydrates raise the level of a chemical in the brain called serotonin. Serotonin elevates moods and regulates sleep.**

---

Your daily diet should contain at least 40% complex carbohydrates, less than 20% protein, and less than 20% fat. During your premenstrual period, you may increase your complex carbohydrate intake and reduce that of protein, for protein may interfere with serotonin synthesis.

Crucifers such as broccoli, cauliflower, cabbage and Brussels sprouts are rich in dietary indoles, which are excellent in removing the excessive hormones mentioned above. Broccoli is also rich in absorbable calcium, which is very helpful in strengthening the bones.

### Herbal Therapy:

Most people who suffer from a severe case of PMS also have a history of yeast disorders and drug, alcohol or nicotine addiction. It is important, therefore, to cleanse the accumulated toxins in the body in order for it to function properly. Focus of cleansing depends on the symptoms of each individual. Usually, it is important to cleanse the blood and digestive tract. In addition, herbal formulas for removing excessive estrogen, progesterone and prolactin should be considered.

### Exercise:

Exercise is particularly helpful with PMS because it generates endorphins, a morphine from within. Endorphins is an opium-like, natural substance which reduces pain and gives a calm, high feeling (without the use of drugs)! Again, don't wait until you are in the middle of PMS to exercise. Do 30 minutes of slow walking every day! This type of exercise will improve your blood circulation and thus reduce the tendency of water retention and muscle aches. The heavy feeling and cramps in your pelvic area can also be reduced or eliminated. Regular exercise can also strengthen the muscle tone in your lower abdomen and thus increase the tolerance for pain or discomfort. A side benefit is that it also helps you become a better lover when you have tight, instead of loose, muscles! And, remember, slow walking is free of charge! What are you waiting for?

### Hands-On Healing:

Hands-on healing techniques such as therapeutic touch and gentle chiropractic adjustment known as craniosacral technique can be very soothing during the onset of PMS. If you feel too uncomfortable to have anyone touch you while experiencing severe cramps, just put your hand(s) on the area that is cramping, such as the lower abdomen or hip areas. The healing energy in your own hands can reduce the cramps and give some relief from pain. You can do this lying down or while you are sitting up, such as while driving.

### *Stress Management:*

Women who are under heavy emotional stress often suffer from more PMS. Whether you agree or not, your body and mind affect each other at all times. Emotional stress can cause all kinds of physical problems including PMS. Remember, all physical illnesses have symbolic meanings. PMS involves the female reproductive system. It requires the examination of emotional issues concerning one's femininity. A woman with a positive self-image usually takes good care of herself and does not give PMS a chance to creep in or sustain itself.

### *Sexercise:*

The Chinese have long believed that if a young woman has PMS, she will grow out of it after she is married. Why? Sexercise!

> **Sex is the best remedy for PMS. Good sex increases self-esteem and improves blood circulation. When you enjoy a good quality and quantity of sex with the right partner, you feel loved and energized.**

Women who suffer from PMS or menopause usually are sexually inactive whether they are married or not. Sexual desire and potency do not have to decline with age. Some of my clients enjoy frequent sex (at least three or four times a week) in their 80s!  You are never too old or too tired for sex!  Remember two principles: 1) you either use it or lose it; and 2) practice makes perfect!   When you learn to enjoy sex on a regular basis, you will learn to enjoy being female.  ***When you enjoy being female or being who you are, chances are you will say goodbye to PMS!***

# Part VII

# Bibliography

# Bibliography

Badgley, L., Healing AIDS Naturally, Human Energy Press, San Bruno, CA, 1987.

Bischko, J., An Introduction to Acupunture, Heinrich Schreck, Maikammer, West-Germany, 1978.

Braly, J., Dr. Braly's Optimum Health Program, Times Books, New York, New York, 1985.

Chen, J. F., Personal conversation on May 19, 1991.

Cheng, X. (Ed.), Chinese Acupuncture and Moxibustion, Foreign Language Press, Beijing, China, 1990.

Chen, Y. and Deng, L., Essentials of Contemporary Chinese Acupunturists' Clinical Experiences, Foreign Languages Press, Beijing, China, 1989.

Clark, H. R., The Cure for All Cancers, ProMotion Publishing, San Diego, CA, 1993.

Corsini, R. J. and Contributors (2nd Ed.), Current Psychotherapies, F. E. Peacock, Itasca, IL, Publishers, 1979.

Cousins, N., Anatomy of an Illness, Bantam Books, New York, New York, 1979.

Crook, W. G., Chronic Fatigue Syndrome and the Yeast Connection, Professional Books, Jackson, Tennessee, 1992.

Crook, W. G., The Yeast Connection (3rd Ed.), Professional Books, Jackson, Tennessee, 1986.

De Schepper, L. Peak Immunity, Luc De Schepper, Santa Monica, CA, 1989.

Doll R. and Peto, R. The Causes of Cancer, Oxford University Press, New York, New York, 1981.

Erickson, M. H. and Rossi, E. L. Hypnotherapy: An Exploratory Casebook, Irvington, New York, New York, 1979.

Feltman, J. and Editors of Prevention Magazine, Hands-On-Healing, Rodale Press, Emmaus, PA, 1989.

Finnegan, J., Yeast Disorders, Elysian Arts, Los Altos, CA, 1987.

Foley, D., Nechas E. and Editors of Prevention Magazine, Women's Encyclopedia of Health and Emotional Healing, Rodale Press, Emmaus, PA, 1993.

Hay, L. L., Heal Your Body, Hay House, Santa Monica, CA, 1982.

Krieger D., The Therapeutic Touch, Prentice Hall, Inc., Englewood Cliffs, NJ, 1979.

Levy, S. M., Behavior and Cancer, Jossey-Bass Publishers, San Francisco, CA, 1985.

Larkin, D. M., "Therapeutic Suggestion." Chapter in Zahourek, R.P. (Ed.), Clinical Hypnosis and Therapeutic Suggestion in Nursing, Grune & Stratton, New York, New York, 1985.

Livingston-Wheeler, V. and Addeo, E. G., The Conquest of Cancer, Franklin Watts, New York, New York, 1984.

Maynard, J. E., Chiropractic: Healing Hands, Jonorm Publishers, Mobile, Alabama, 1977.

McDougall, J. A. and McDougall, M. A., The McDougall Plan, New Century Publishers, Picataway, New Jersey, 1983.

Nourse, A. E., Your Immune System, Franklin Watts, New York, New York, 1989.

Perls, F. S., Gestalt Therapy Verbatim, Real People Press, Moab, Utah, 1969.

Perls, F. S., and Clements C. C.: "Acting Out vs. Acting Through" in Stevens, J. O. (Ed.): Gestalt Is, Real People Press, Moab, Utah, 1975.

Pope, L., "Research Ties Smog to Cancer." Los Angeles Daily News, October 25, 1991, p. 14.

Robbins, J., Diet for a New America, Stillpoint Publishing, Walpole, NH, 1987.

Rose, E., Lady of Gray: Healing Candida (2nd Ed.), Butterfly Publishing Co., Santa Monica, CA, 1985.

Satir, V., Conjoint Family Therapy, Science and Behavior Books, Inc., Palo Alto, CA, 1967.

Schwartz, M. S. and Associates, Biofeedback: A Practitioner's Guide, The Guilford Press, New York, New York, 1987.

Siegel, B. S., Peace, Love and Healing, Harper & Row Publishers, New York, New York, 1989.

Spiegel, H., "An Eyeroll Test for Hypnotizability." American Journal of Clinical Hypnosis, 15, 25-28.

Stoff, J. A. and Pellegrino, C. R., Chronic Fatigue Syndrome, Harper Perennial, New York, New York, 1992.

Talbot, M., Your Past Lives, Harmony Books, New York, New York, 1987.

Teeguarden, I. M., Acupressure Way of Health: Jin Shin Do, Japan Publications, Inc., New York, New York, 1978.

Tien, J. L., Healthy and Tasty: Anti-Yeast Cooking, Infinite Success International Publishing House, Las Vegas, Nevada, 1997.

Tien, J. L., <u>Being the Best You Can Be -- A Practical Guide for Harmony and Prosperity</u>, (a book and six cassette tapes), Infinite Success International Publishing House, Las Vegas, Nevada, 1996.

Tien, J. L., "Chinese Herbal Therapy for Pain Management." Paper presented at the American Academy of Pain Management Annual Convention, Dallas, Texas, September 15, 1995.

Tien, J. L., "Chinese Herbs -- How to Get the Best Results." <u>Whole Life Times</u>, November, 1994, p. 59.

Tien, J. L., "Understanding & Healing Your Pain -- Using a Non-intrusive, Non-drug Approach." <u>COSI - L.A. Community Magazine</u>, October, 1994, p. 20.

Tien, J. L., "Kids Who Can't Sit Still--Attention Deficit Disorder." <u>Whole Life Times</u>, October, 1993, p. 16.

Tien, J. L., "Body, Mind and Spirit Connection: Nursing Challenge for 1990's." Paper presented at the 20th Quadrennial International Congress of Nurses Conference, Madrid, Spain, June 24, 1993.

Tien, J. L., "Attention Deficit Disorder." <u>Daily News</u>, Monday, June 7, 1993, L. A. Life, p. 27.

Tien-Hyatt, J. L., "Conquer Stress -- And Find Peace in the New Year." <u>Whole Life Times</u>, January, 1993, p. 39.

Tien-Hyatt, J. L., "Weight Problems and Yeast Disorders." <u>Family Living</u>, July, 1992, p. 45.

Tien-Hyatt, J. L., "Are You Sick and Tired of Being Sick and Tired?" <u>Fraternal Order of Police Journal</u>, summer, 1992, pp. 47-49.

Tien-Hyatt, J. L., "Too Pooped to Pop -- Conquering Chronic Fatigue Syndrome." <u>Whole Life Times</u>, January, 1992, p. 15.

Tien-Hyatt, J. L., "Boost Your Immunity and Vitality." <u>Family Living</u>, Dec., 1991, p.51.

Tien-Hyatt, J. L., "Candida: It Does Anything But Sweeten Your Life." <u>Whole Life Times</u>, July 1991, p. 27.

Tien-Hyatt, J. L., "Manage Your Weight Effectively by Nourishing Your Body and Mind." <u>Family Living</u>, June, 1991, p. 60.

Tien-Hyatt, J. L., "The Holistic Approach to Pain Management: A Preliminary Study." Paper presented at the 1987 Annual Sigma Theta Tau, Gamma Tau Research Conference, Duarte, California, March 20, 1987.

Tien-Hyatt, J. L., "Self-perceptions of Aging Across Cultures: Myth or Reality?" <u>International Journal of Aging and Human Development</u>, Vol. 24(2), 1986-87 (Research paper).

Tien-Hyatt, J. L., "Holistic Mental Health Nursing: Combining Psychological Counseling, Acupressure and Hypnotherapy." Paper presented at the Third International Congress of Psychiatric Nursing, London, England, September 23, 1986.

Tien, J. L., "Home Remedies as Alternative Health Care: A Cross Culture Study." Paper presented at the 18th Quadrennial International Congress of Nurses Conference, Tel Aviv, Israel, June 19, 1985.

Tien, J. L. "Cultural Variation in Life Satisfaction for the Elderly: East and West." Abstract, The Gerontologist, Vol. 3, Special Issue, p. 296, October, 1983 (Research Report).

Tien, J. L., "Self-perceptions of Aging and Family Networks: A Cross Cultural Study." Abstract, Southwest Anthropological Association Program and Abstracts, p. 94, April, 1982 (Research Report).

Tien, J. L., A Descriptive Cross-cultural Study on Factors Associated with Self-perceptions of Aging among Anglo-Americans, Chinese Americans and Chinese in Taiwan, Dissertation, University of California, San Francisco, 1981.

Trowbridge, J. and Walker, M., The Yeast Syndrome, Bantam Books, New York, New York, 1986.

Truss, C. O., The Missing Diagnosis, The Missing Diagnosis Inc., Birmingham, Alabama, 1985.

Quillin, P., Healing Nutrients, Vintage Books, New York, New York, 1989.

Wade, C., Eat Away Illness, Parker Publishibg Company, West Nyack, New York, 1986.

Weiss, B. L., Many Lives, Many Masters, Simon & Schuster, New York, New Yor, 1988.

Woolger, R. J., Other Lives, Other Selves, Bantam Books, New York, New York, 1988.

Willner, R. E., Deadly Deception, Peltec Publishing Co., Inc., Boca Raton, FL, 1994.

Willner, R. E., The Cancer Solution, Peltec Publishing Co., Inc., Boca Raton, FL, 1994.

Yalom, I., The Theory and Practice of Group Psychotherapy, Basic Books, New York, New York, 1988.

Zahourek, R. P. (Ed.), Clinical Hypnosis and Therapeutic Suggestion in Nursing, Grune & Stratton, New York, New York, 1985.

# Part VIII

# About the Author

# About the Author

## CURRICULUM VITAE
(Summary of Selected Professional Activities)

Name: **Juliet L. Tien, D. N. Sc., M. S. N., B. S. N., R. N., C. S.**
Address: 12021 Wilshire Blvd., Ste. 197
W. Los Angeles, CA 90025
Telephone: (310) 477-5302    Fax: (310) 477-4271    E-Mail: DrJ@drjshealthnet.com
California License Numbers: P188 & RN 252774

## EDUCATION:

Doctorate in Nursing Science in Mental Health, Family Health and Psychogerontology, University of California, San Francisco, 1981.
Master's in Nursing Science (M. S. N.) in Psychiatric/Mental Health Nursing, Boston College, Massachusetts, 1973.
Bachelor in Nursing Science (B. S. N.) in Basic Nursing, National Taiwan University School of Nursing, 1970.

## SPECIAL TRAINING AND CERTIFICATION:

- Hypnotherapy, Chinese Herbal Therapy, Nutritional Counseling and Acupressure
- State of California BRN Provider for Continuing Education Programs
- Nationally Certified Clinical Specialist (C. S.) in Psychiatric/Mental Health Nursing.

## SPECIALTIES:

Counseling for Addiction Control, Pain Management, Post-traumatic Stress Disorder, Domestic Violence and Victims of Crime, Sexual Abuse/Harassment, Attention Deficit Disorder (ADD), Chronic Fatigue Syndrome (CFS), Permanent Weight Control, and Relationships.

## GRANTS AND AWARDS:

1984-87    Ethnic Mental Health Nurse Specialist Training Grant, National Institute of Mental Health (Grant #: 1 To 1 MH 18112).
1986    Minority Nursing Leadership Conference Grant, California Office of Statewide Health Planning and Development (Grant #: 85-G0054).
1984-85    Institute of American Culture Research Grant (Attitudes Toward Divorce and Divorce Adjustment among Asian Americans).

| | |
|---|---|
| 1983-85 Asian | UCLA Academic Senate Research Grant (Divorce Among Anglo and Americans). |
| 1982-83 among | UCLA Academic Senate Research Grant (Self-perceptions of Aging Japanese Americans). |
| 1981-82 | UCLA Academic Senate Research Grant (A Cross-cultural Study on Self-perceptions of Aging and Associated Factors). |
| 1979-81 | Title II Traineeship Grant (Grant #: 2 All Nu00289-04). |
| 1978-79 | NIMH Traineeship Grant (Grant #: 5 To 3-MH13621-05). |

## PROFESSIONAL EXPERIENCE:

| | |
|---|---|
| 1996- Present | Cable Television Producer: "The Holistic Approach to Health and Success." |
| 1996- Present | Motivational speaker at various institutions including Daniel Freeman Hospital and Medical Center at Inglewood and Marina del Rey, California. |
| 1995- Present | Founding President, Infinite Success International (An International Network Marketing Company for Continuing Education programs and Chinese herbal products). |
| 1989- Present | Founding President, Dr. J's Health Institute and Professional Weight Management Centers, Brentwood and Woodland Hills, California (Chinese herbal therapy, nutritional therapy, psychological counseling, hypnotherapy, acupressure, mental health consultation and continuing education (locally, nationally, and internationally). |
| 1990 | Consultant, Whittier Hospital and Medical Center, Cross-cultural Health Care, Whittier, California. |
| 1987-1989 | Founding President, The Institute of Holistic Health, Santa Monica, California. |
| 1982-1987 | Consultant, Sigma Theta Tau, Gamma Tau Chapter, Cultural Research, Los Angeles, California. |
| 1981-87 | Asst. Professor and Principal Investigator/Project Director, Ethnic Mental Health Nurse Specialist Program, UCLA School of Nursing, Los Angeles, California. |
| 1982-84 | Founding President, Chinese American Nurses Association, USA. |
| 1982 | Consultant, Formosan Hope Line, Rosemead, California. |
| 1982 | Consultant, Taiwan Provincial Kaohsiung Mental Hospital, Kaohsiung, Taiwan. |
| 1981 | Consultant, Kaohsiung Medical Center, School of Nursing, Kaohsiung, Taiwan. |
| 1981 | Consultant, The Taipei College of Nursing and Teaching Hospital, Taipei, Taiwan. |
| 1981 | Consultant, Hong Kong Politechs, Department of Social Services, Hong Kong. |
| 1980 | In-service Educator, Self-Help for the Elderly, San Francisco, California. |
| 1968-80 | Psychological counselor, staff nurse, nursing supervisor, Director of Nurses in various counseling centers, hospitals and long-term care |

facilities.

## SELECTED PUBLICATIONS:

Tien, J. L., Healthy and Tasty: Anti-Yeast Cooking, Infinite Success International Publishing House, Las Vegas, Nevada, 1997.

Tien, J. L., Being the Best You Can Be -- A Practical Guide for Harmony and Prosperity, (a book and six cassette tapes), Infinite Success International Publishing House, Las Vegas, Nevada, 1996.

Tien, J. L., "Chinese Herbal Therapy for Pain Management." Paper presented at the American Academy of Pain Management Annual Convention, Dallas, Texas, September 15, 1995.

Tien, J. L., "Chinese Herbs -- How to Get the Best Results." Whole Life Times, November, 1994, p. 59.

Tien, J. L., "Understanding & Healing Your Pain -- Using a Non-intrusive, Non-drug Approach." COSI - L.A. Community Magazine, October, 1994, p. 20.

Tien, J. L., "Kids Who Can't Sit Still--Attention Deficit Disorder." Whole Life Times, October, 1993, p. 16.

Tien, J. L., "Body, Mind and Spirit Connection: Nursing Challenge for 1990's." Paper presented at the 20th Quadrennial International Congress of Nurses Conference, Madrid, Spain, June 24, 1993.

Tien, J. L., "Attention Deficit Disorder." Daily News, Monday, June 7, 1993, L. A. Life, p. 27.

Tien-Hyatt, J. L., "Conquer Stress -- And Find Peace in the New Year." Whole Life Times, January, 1993, p. 39.

Tien-Hyatt, J. L., "Weight Problems and Yeast Disorders." Family Living, July, 1992, p. 45.

Tien-Hyatt, J. L., "Are You Sick and Tired of Being Sick and Tired?" Fraternal Order of Police Journal, summer, 1992, pp. 47-49.

Tien-Hyatt, J. L., "Too Pooped to Pop -- Conquering Chronic Fatigue Syndrome." Whole Life Times, January, 1992, p. 15.

Tien-Hyatt, J. L., "Boost Your Immunity and Vitality." Family Living, Dec., 1991, p. 51.

Tien-Hyatt, J. L., "Candida: It Does Anything But Sweeten Your Life." Whole Life Times, July, 1991, p. 27.

Tien-Hyatt, J. L., "Manage Your Weight Effectively by Nourishing Your Body and Mind." Family Living, June, 1991, p. 60.

Tien-Hyatt, J. L., "Mental Health Considerations Across Cultures." Chapter in Varcarotis, E.N. (Ed.) Foundations of Psychiatric Mental Health Nursing, W.B. Saunders Co., 1990, pp. 65-82.

Tien-Hyatt, J. L., "Keying on the Unique Care Needs of Asian Clients," Journal of Nursing and Health Care, Vol. 8, No. 5, pp. 269-271, May, 1987 (Article).

Tien-Hyatt, J. L., "The Holistic Approach to Pain Management: A Preliminary Study." Paper presented at the 1987 Annual Sigma Theta Tau, Gamma Tau Research Conference, Duarte, California, March 20, 1987.

Tien-Hyatt, J. L., "Self-perceptions of Aging Across Cultures: Myth or Reality?" International Journal of Aging and Human Development, Vol. 24(2), 1986-87 (Research paper).

Tien-Hyatt, J. L., "Holistic Mental Health Nursing: Combining Psychological Counseling,, Acupressure and Hypnotherapy." Paper presented at the Third International Congress of Psychiatric Nursing, London, England, September 23, 1986.

Tien-Hyatt, J. L., "Leadership Qualities: Determinants of Positive Self-Image and Career Success for Minority Nursing Leadership: Past and Future, sponsored by the State of California, Office of Statewide Health Planning and Development, San Francisco, California, May 16, 1986.

Tien, J. L. and Johnson, H. L., "Black Mental Health Client's Preference for Therapists: A New Look at an Old Issue." International Journal of Social Psychiatry, Vol. 31, No. 4, pp. 258-266, Winter, 1985 (Research Paper).

Tien, J. L., "Divorce Adjustments Across Three Cultures: Implications for Preventive Mental Health." Paper presented at the 1985 Biennial World Federation for Mental Health Conference, Brighton, England, July 18, 1985.

Tien, J. L., "Home Remedies as Alternative Health Care: A Cross Culture Study." Paper presented at the 18th Quadrennial International Congress of Nurses Conference, Tel Aviv, Israel, June 19, 1985.

Tien, J. L., "Do Asians Need Less Medication? Issues in Clinical Assessment -- A Nursing Perspective." Journal of Psychosocial Nursing, Vol. 22, pp. 19-22, December, 1984 (Article).

Tien, J. L., "Toward a Theoretical Model for Cross-Cultural Studies of Aging." Abstract, the Proceedings of the 17th Annual Communicating Nursing Research Conference, May, 1984.

Tien, J. L., "Cultural Variation in Life Satisfaction for the Elderly: East and West." Abstract, The Gerontologist, Vol. 3, Special Issue, p. 296, October, 1983 (Research Report).

Tien, J. L., "Self-perceptions of Aging and Family Networks: A Cross Cultural Study." Abstract, Southwest Anthropological Association Program and Abstracts, p. 94, April, 1982 (Research Report).

Abu-Saad H., Kayser-Jones J. and Tien, J. L., "Asian-American Nursing Students in the United States." Journal of Nursing Education, Vol. 21, No. 7, pp. 11-15, September, 1982 (Research Paper).

Tien, J. L., "Surviving Graduate Nursing Programs in the United States -- A Personal Account." Journal of Nursing Education, Vol. 21, pp. 42-44, September, 1982 (Article).

## PRESENTATIONS:

Since 1968, has made over 180 presentations in the area of cross-culture mental health, holistic health, yeast disorders, Chronic Fatigue Syndrome (CFS), permanent weight control, domestic violence and victims of crime, sexual harassment, Post-traumatic Stress Disorder, Attention Deficit Disorder (ADD), Chinese herbal therapy, natural remedies for diabetes, and holistic approach to pain management in local, national and international conferences.

## THESIS AND DISSERTATION COMMITTEES:

Served as a chairperson or committee member on more than 15 Master Thesis or Doctoral Dissertation Committees at UCLA and other universities.

## MEDIA APPEARANCES:

Since 1981, has appeared as a host or guest in over 300 radio talk shows or televised programs focusing on the holistic approach to health and success. Examples: from 1987 to 1994, the host of radio talk show on holistic health on KIEV, KFOX and KWNK. In 1994, interviewed on KFWB, KMAX and KMPC, Los Angeles, California regarding the holistic approach to earthquake flus and blues. In 1995, interviewed on KCTV, Santa Barbara, California regarding the holistic approach to health and success. Currently, a producer of cable television programs entitled, "The Holistic Approach to Health and Success." Since July 1996, has produced over 20 televised talks hows for Public Access programs.

## HONORS:

1986        The Most Outstanding Professional of the Year, awarded by Chinese Joint Professionals.

1982 - Present  Member of Sigma Theta Tau, International Nursing Honor Society

1971        Youth Model, awarded by China Youth Corp.

# Part IX

## Services, Chinese Herbal Formulas, and Organic, Vegetarian Food
available at
### Dr. J's Health Institute
and
### Dr. J's Healthy & Tasty Restaurant

# Dr. J's Health Institute

**11819 Wilshire Blvd., Ste. 213**
**West Los Angeles, CA 90025**
**Tel: (310) 477-5302    Fax: (310) 477-4271    Web Site: www.drjshealthnet.com**

*Balance your body, mind and spirit to maximize your energy, mental clarity, productivity and accomplishments by using a combination of the following:*

1) **Chinese Herbal Formulas** for detoxifying and regenerating your body.
2) **Anti-Yeast Nutritional Program** for nourishing your body and starving your enemies (yeast and parasites).
3) **Spiritual Psychotherapy** for relinquishing your deep, negative emotions and increasing your receptivity for an abundance of love and resources.
4) **Past-Life Therapy** for releasing your spiritual trauma and starting your life on a clean slate.

---

## *Our Private-Brand Chinese Herbal Formulas:*

**Yeast-Para Control:** Cleanse yeast and parasites and relieve yourself of the burden of feeding an "extended family." You will see evidence in your toilet (e.g., debris of yeast, and eggs and bodies of parasites) in a few days!

**Cleansing-Balance Tea:** Cleanse your liver and kidneys, and strengthen your immune, digestive, respiratory and cardio-vascular systems. Can also improve your eyesight. You'll enjoy this caffeine-free herbal tea all day and all year round.

**Female Vitality:** A combination of high quality and absorbable vitamins, minerals and Chinese herbs to nourish your body and balance your hormonal system. Excellent for increasing your energy and mental clarity, and alleviating PMS and menopausal symptoms.

**Male Vitality:** A combination of high quality and absorbable vitamins, minerals and Chinese herbs to nourish your body and balance your hormonal system. Excellent for increasing your energy, mental clarity, and sexual potency, and controlling prostate inflammation.

**Weight Control System:**

    **Herbal Cocktail:** A blend of high quality grains, fibers, Chinese herbs and digestive enzymes to nourish your body, curb your junk-food (especially sugar) craving. Excellent with breakfast or as an in-between-meal drink.

    **Fitness Regular:** A unique formula designed to: prevent your body from absorbing unwanted fats from the food you eat, remove fats from your body (like "Pac Man"), improve your cardio-vascular function, and balance your blood sugar, blood pressure and cholesterol. Excellent for athletes, people who want to lose weight, or those who simply want to remain trim!

    **Fitness Plus:** A powerful formula designed to burn the existing fats in your body and turn them into energy. It strengthens your thyroid gland and improves your metabolism.

*\*\*\* Please note: Several formulas, such as **Yeast-Para Control**, **Cleansing-Balance Tea**, **Male Vitality** and **Female Vitality** are also beneficial to your pets. The general rule for pet intake is one capsule for every 10 pounds. For example, if your dog weighs 50 pounds, give it five (5) capsules of **Yeast-Para Control**, and five (5) capsules of **Male** or **Female Vitality**. Also, feed it with one (1) cup of **Cleansing-Balance Tea** per day. You may open the capsules and mix the contents with pet food, or have your pets swallow the capsules by using the following procedure: 1) holding their mouths open, 2) dropping the capsules into their throats, 3) closing their mouths, and 4) rubbing their throats gently to help the capsules go down the digestive tract.*

## Testimonials from Our Happy Clients:

*I saw Dr. J briefly for consultation 10 years ago and I quickly "ran away" because I thought her holistic treatment was too radical. Ten years later I came back to see her because I was overweight and I had a lump in my breast. After about six weeks of sticking to her anti-yeast nutritional program, taking weight control formulas (including **Herbal Cocktail**, **Fitness Regular** and **Fitness Plus**), **Yeast-Para Control** and the **Cleansing-Balance Tea**, I lost 11 pounds and three inches around my waistline. Most of all, when I went to my physician for a scheduled surgery to remove the lump, it disappeared! No surgery was needed!*     -- Peggy K. Teacher, Los Angeles, California

*I have been overweight all my life. This is the first time I'm able to drop 47 pounds in three months and keep it off using Dr. J's anti-yeast nutritional program and **Weight Control Herbs**. I also enjoy a lot of energy and mental clarity.*
    -- Carol H., R. N., Ventura, California

*I had yeast and parasitic infection symptoms from head to toe. After being on **Yeast-Para Control** and **Female Vitality** formulas and the **Cleansing-Balance Tea** for three months, plus releasing negative emotions through private consultation with Dr. J, my symptoms of allergies, sinus headaches, constipation, bloating, fatigue, PMS, depression, anemia and sugar craving had all dissipated. I now feel like a new person!*
    -- Margie, L., Secretary, Santa Monica, California

*I was a diabetic for more than 10 years. I was insulin dependent and overweight and had no energy. Dr. J's **Weight Control System**, **Yeast-Para Control**, **Male Vitality**, the **Cleansing-Balance Tea** and the anti-yeast nutritional program had created a new life for me. In two months, I was able to reduce my insulin to one-third of my previous dosage. I have also lost 15 pounds and dropped my cholesterol by 51 points. After one year, I am totally off medication for diabetes! I now have much more energy. I highly recommend the program!*     -- Bob F., Realtor, Glendale, California

*I had been asthmatic and dependent on cortisone inhalers since I could remember. After I took Dr. J's **Yeast-Para Control** formula and the **Cleansing-Balance Tea**, plus made a commitment to her anti-yeast nutritional program, for the first time in 20 years, I do not need to use the inhaler!* -- Sue, T, Salesperson, Culver City, California

*As a personal trainer, I have always tried different herbal products and looked for safe weight control products for my clients. I'm pleased to find that Dr. J's **Weight Control System** is very cost-effective. The products reduce fat, improve overall muscle tone and increase energy. The Yeast-Para Control formula is a great product for clearing age-old mucous and smooth elimination. It works well with the **Weight Control System** to help my clients achieve an optimal level of functioning!* -- Mary A., Fitness Trainer, Sherman Oaks, California

*For several years I have experimented with many diets trying to lose 10 pounds. I would lose a few pounds initially, but then the weight loss stopped. I got on Dr. J's **Weight Control System**, and to my surprise, I easily lost 11 pounds in four weeks! My total weight loss is 15 pounds after strictly following her plan, and I feel great! Dr. J's program is a healthy alternative to fad diets that just don't work. Changing eating habits is never easy, but a commitment to a healthy lifestyle is helpful.* -- Fran B., R. N., Thousand Oaks, California

*I'm very pleased with Dr. J's **Weight Control System**. As a physician, I was skeptical about these herbs in the beginning. But once I got on the program, I lost 3 inches and 14 pounds in one month. I have lost a total of 20 pounds and I'm now on the maintenance program. I have a lot of energy and stamina. I don't need to snack in between meals. Even when I'm hungry, I'm easily satisfied after I eat. I don't eat a big portion of meals like I did before. The program is also easy to follow and cost-effective comparing with other programs I know.* -- Jack J., M. D., Beverly Hills, California

*I had herpes. The frequent outbreaks had precluded me from being sexually active. I was also told by my previous physician that I had to live with this "sexual and emotional handicap" for the rest of my life. I was angry, depressed and irritable. After I took Dr. J's **Yeast-Para Control**, **Male Vitality**, and **Cleansing Balance Tea** for three months, and consulted Dr. J periodically to learn how to reduce stress, the symptoms subsided. As long as I continue to treat myself regularly according to Dr. J's instructions and take the herbs, I am symptom free and a happy camper again!* -- Albert G, Film Maker, Hollywood, California

*I suffered from candidiasis for years. I was underweight, lethargic, bloated and prone to kidney and bladder infections. I also had skin rash all over my body. After taking **Yeast-Para Control**, **Female Vitality** and the **Cleansing-Balance Tea** and following Dr. J's anti-yeast nutritional program, I gained 7 pounds in two months. My skin is now clearing up. I rarely feel bloated unless I eat the wrong kind of food (yeast favorite food) again. I haven't had any episode of kidney or bladder infections since I started the program. I also have a lot more energy!* -- Ellen R., Actress, New York, New York

*I usually have a problem with portion control and sluggish metabolism. One day after I started the Dr. J's herbal **Weight Control System**, I felt like something immediately "jump-started" my system -- sort of tingled all over. I got a terrible headache, my face broke out, and I couldn't sleep for half of the night, but I was happy because I knew it was a battle of toxins vs. purity! Of course, all these cleansing symptoms dissipated in the next few days! My appetite is under control and I lost 12 pounds in one month. This is powerful stuff!*                          Kay U. Retired Executive, Albuquergue, New Mexico

*I was searching all over for a holistic doctor to treat my Chronic Fatigue Syndrome and yeast infections. I took several anti-fungal drugs in the past few years with short-term effects. Finally, I met Dr. J while I was vacationing (and searching) in California. Her common-sensed anti-yeast nutritional program is easy to follow, and her herbal formulas work immediately -- I am still seeing the debris of yeast and eggs and bodies of parasites when I do "toilet watching" as Dr. J instructed. The combination of **Yeast-Para Control**, **Cleansing Balance Tea**, **Herbal Cocktail** and **Male Vitality** has changed my life! Her deep emotional releasing technique has also helped me remove "mental toxins." I now have more positive attitudes and better outlooks on life. It's wonderful to be able to enjoy life again!*                          -- Jay R., Businessman, Columbus, Ohio

*I did not believe that I had long-term yeast and parasitic infections until I saw the evidence in my toilet and menstrual blood clogs-- eggs of parasites and bodies of various kinds of yeast and worms! It was so gross, and yet I was happy that my enemies were out of my system after I was on Dr. J's **Yeast-Para Control** formula and **Cleansing-Balance Tea** for just a few weeks. It is not easy to follow Dr. J's anti-yeast nutritional program in this part of the country, but when I do, I see results! I have been taking her herbal formulas religiously and following the instructions in her books to reduce stress. My life will be so much easier when Dr. J opens her restaurants and health food markets in this area.*                          -- Demi, F., Housewife, Wilson, North Carolina

*My dog was diagnosed with "invasive Cancer" -- carcinoma, last September. The veterinarian did not think he was going to live too long. He was loosing hair and appetite, and was bleeding rectally. He has been on Dr. J's **Male Vitality, Yeast-Para Control and Cleansing-Balance Tea** for six months now. His hair looks very healthy and he eats well. His rectal bleeding has also been reduced substantially. When I took him back to see the vet a few days ago, she could not believe that he lived and looked so well! Even though she did not believe in herbs, she commented, "I cannot quarrel with the results!"*                          -- Rhonda A., Office Manager, Middleburg, Pennsylvania

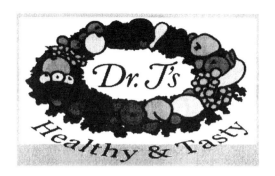

## *Organic Vegetarian*
**Fast Food Restaurant**

**1303 Westwood Blvd.**
**Los Angeles, CA 90024**
**(Two blocks south of Wilshire Blvd., near UCLA)**

**Tel. (310) 477-2721     FAX. (310) 477-8841**
Website: www.drjshealthnet.com

*\* Hot Meals \*Soups \*Sandwiches \*Snacks*
*\*Beverages \*Desserts \*Herbs*
*\*Freshly Packed Frozen-Food*

All of our recipes are developed by Dr. Juliet Tien (Dr. J), a renowned author and television celebrity, based on her personal and professional experiences treating yeast and parasitic infections for more than three decades.  Every item on our menu is created with a great deal of thought and care!

**Business Hours:** Mon.- Sat.: 11 a.m. – 9 p.m.
(Lunch Buffet: 11 a.m. – 5 p.m., Dinner: 5 – 9 p.m.)
## *We Cater and Deliver*

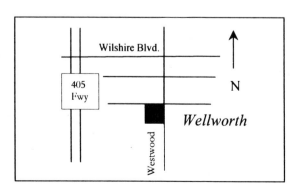

# Why Are We Healthier than the Rest?

1. **We use no sugar, dairy, wheat, yeast, alcohol, caffeine, MSG, nor chemicals in our cooking.** Most other restaurants use a lot of sugar and wheat that may cause you allergic reactions including fatigue, bloating, mucous, muscle aches and mind fog.

2. **Our Yeast-Free vegetarian cuisine is based on our ten-year track record providing freshly-packed frozen food to our clients.** After thousands of clients rid themselves of health problems including allergies, fatigue, weight gain, or weight loss, they requested that we open a chain of hot food restaurants.

3. **We use olive or canola oil in our cooking. These oils contain the lowest concentration of saturated fats.** Your body needs good fats to get rid of bad fats.

4. **We are dedicated to using only the finest organic ingredients.** Non-organic produce is loaded with pesticides that are harmful to your health.

5. **Our food is vegetarian.** Most meats and fish are loaded with antibiotics, growth hormones or preservatives that are detrimental to your health.

6. **To suit your busy schedule, we provide you with fast food in a buffet style.** When you're on the run, fast and healthy food is invaluable!

7. **We use a high heat, fast, stir-fry cooking method that eliminates the yeast and parasites on raw foods, but still maintains the maximum amount of life energy and nutrients of the foods.** For most people, raw foods are difficult to digest. Raw foods also contain a lot of yeast and parasite eggs. On the contrary, canned foods are cooked to death, and have little or no nutritional value. We provide you with the happy medium!

8. **We wash our vegetables thoroughly before cooking.** An extra step to reduce or eliminate yeast, eggs of parasites, bacteria, and viruses on the produce.

9. **We incorporate the best of yin and yang, macrobiotic, and Ayurveda principles in our cooking.** Our food gives you a good nutritional balance based on ancient and contemporary knowledge of how food leads you to good health.

10. **Nobody has delicious baked goods and snacks like we do -- completely free of yeast, dairy, wheat, eggs, sugar, salt, and chemicals.** Compare and you will notice and enjoy the difference!

11. **For your better health, we use only clean, disposable utensils.** One additional healthy benefit for you!

12. **Our food is not only healthy, but also tasty!** Try it, and you 'll be amazed and pleased!

# Testimonials from Our Happy Customers

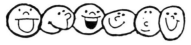

*I have been eating at* **Dr. J's Healthy & Tasty Restaurant** *several times a week since it's opening. I have noticed that I don't feel bloated after I eat. I also don't need to take a nap like I used to after lunch. I enjoy the taste and the benefits of the food!*
-- Aaron B., Businessman, Westwood, Southern California

*I was a meat eater. After tasting Dr. J's Vegie Chicken Nuggets, Vegie Chicken Balls, Vegie Ham, Vegie Fish and Vegie Shrimp, I no longer have the desire to eat animal meats. I now look forward to receiving the delivery of hot and frozen food every week!*
-- Sam O., Retired Postman, West Los Angeles, California

*I am so glad that I can order Dr. J's healthy snacks through the mail now. A scoop of* **Herbal Cocktail** *in a cup of hot* **Cleansing-Balance Tea** *and a sugar- and wheat-free oat bran cookie or Supersnack in the late afternoon is just like heaven! It takes away my sugar craving and gives me the energy I need for the rest of the day. I enjoy cereals and oat bran muffins for breakfast too!*
-- Gladys F., R. N., Seattle, Washington

*It is a blessing in the sky that Dr. J opened her first restaurant in my neighborhood! It has been difficult to find vegetarian restaurants, let alone restaurants serving yeast-free food! The taste, color and fragrance of Dr. J's food are superb! Thanks Dr. J for making my life so much easier by providing really healthy and tasty food!*
-- Roberta C., Businesswoman, Santa Monica, California

*I suffered Irritated Bowel Syndrome for years. The food at Dr. J's Healthy & Tasty Restaurant does wonders for my digestive system! Whenever I eat Dr. J's food, I do not experience bloating or diarrhea like I did before. The food also tastes great. The fish steaks, chicken balls, chicken nuggets, and shrimp are made of soy, but taste better and are healthier than real meats or seafood. Amazing!*
-- David F., M. D., Westwood, Southern California

*Dr. J's organic, vegetarian, fast food restaurant is my lifesaver! My body responds well to food with no sugar, dairy, wheat and yeast. In the past, I had to go through the hassle of shopping and preparing yeast-free food in the midst of my busy schedule. Now, with Dr. J's hot and frozen food, I will not go hungry again!*
-- Susan L., Business Consultant, Beverly Hills, California

*I could go several days without leaving my house when I had to meet a deadline. Dr. J's hot food, sandwiches, snacks, and frozen food have made my life so much easier! I usually "shop" at Dr. J's restaurant once a week and stock up on a week's supply of food. The food satisfies my tummy and improves my mental clarity and productivity. Best of all, the frozen food is portion-controlled and calorie-counted. It keeps my weight down!*
-- Stephen S., Producer and Screenplay Writer, Brentwood, Southern California

# Dr. J's Health Institute
**Mailing Address for placing your order:**
12021 Wilshire Blvd., Ste. 197, W. Los Angeles, CA 90025
Tel. (310) 477-5302     Fax: (310) 477-4271

| Herbal Formulas | Health Benefits | Price | Qty | Subtotal |
|---|---|---|---|---|
| **Weight Control (one-month supply):** | | | | |
| Herbal Cocktail | Weight & Appetite Control; Energy; High Protein Nourishment; Smooth Elimination | $ 33.00 | | |
| Fitness Regular | Weight Control; Building Lean Muscle; Balancing Blood Sugar, Blood Pressure &Cholesterol; Improving Blood Circulation | 50.00 | | |
| Fitness Plus | Weight Control; Fat-burner; Improving Metabolism, Energy, & Mental Clarity | 67.00 | | |
| **Yeast-Para Control** | Yeast & Parasite Control; Immunity; Allergy Control | 25.00 (one bottle for a 10-day supply) 75.00 (three bottles for a one-month supply) | | |
| **Female Vitality** | Hormonal Balance; Energy; Healthy Hair, Nails & Skin | 25.00 (one bottle for a 10-day supply) 75.00 (three bottles for a one-month supply) | | |
| **Male Vitality** | Energy; Healthy Prostate, Hair, Nails and Skin; Sexual Potency | 25.00 (one bottle for a 10-day supply) 75.00 (three bottles for a one-month supply) | | |
| **Cleansing-Balance Tea** | Cleansing and Balancing Liver, Kidneys, Lungs, and Cardio-vascular, Digestive and Immune Systems | 16.00 (one-month supply) | | |
| **Books and Tapes** | | | | |
| **Breaking the Yeast Curse: Food and Unconditional Love for Magic Healing** | Regarded as the "Bible of Health" and "Life-Long Companion" | 17.99 | | |
| **Healthy and Tasty: Dr. J's Anti-Yeast Cooking** | Regarded as the "most simple, effective, and delicious anti-yeast cookbook" | 9.99 | | |
| **Ten-Minute Meditation** | A meditation tape which induces instant relaxation! | 9.99 | | |
| **Being the Best You Can Be: A Practical Guide for Harmony and Prosperity** | A workbook and six (6) cassette tapes designed to improve your outlook on life, interpersonal relationships and financial resources! | 150.00 | | |

**Subtotal:**

Tax (8.25% for California Residents)
Shipping and Handling ($5.00 minimum or 5% if the order is over $100.00)
**Total:**

_____ **Check or Money Order**  _____ **MasterCard or Visa #:** _____

**Expiration Date:** _____  **Card Holder:** _____

**Name:** _____  **Address:** _____

**Telephone Number (_____)** _____